# Freeze-Dried Weight Loss: A Culinary Journey to Health

## Chapter 1: Introduction

In an era marked by the rise of convenience foods and sedentary lifestyles, obesity has reached epidemic proportions, becoming a significant public health concern. The relentless march of this condition has given rise to various health complications, affecting millions of lives worldwide. As waistlines expand and health deteriorates, there's an urgent need for a collective shift toward healthier living.

The obesity epidemic is not just about aesthetics; it's a matter of life and death. Excess weight is associated with a host of chronic diseases, such as diabetes, heart disease, and even certain types of cancer. These conditions diminish our quality of life and can shorten our time on this planet. We all have a stake in addressing this issue, not only for ourselves but for the generations to come.

But the path to better health is not about drastic, unsustainable diets or deprivation. It's about making informed choices, embracing a balanced approach to nutrition, and finding ways to enjoy food without compromising your health. This book explores a unique avenue for achieving weight loss and overall well-being through freeze-dried foods.

While there's no one-size-fits-all solution to this complex problem, we aim to shed light on the potential of freeze-dried foods as a viable and sustainable approach to weight management. Freeze-dried foods offer a bridge between convenience and nutrition, providing a way to enjoy flavorful, nutrient-rich meals while working towards a healthier weight.

In the pages that follow, we'll delve into the science and art of freeze-drying, understanding its unique benefits for weight loss. We'll explore the nutritional value of freeze-dried foods, uncover creative meal planning strategies, and share delicious recipes. From managing portion sizes to curbing cravings, we'll provide practical tips and insights to guide you on your journey to a healthier you.

It's time to take control of your health, tackle the obesity epidemic head-on, and find a sustainable path to weight loss and a healthier lifestyle. Welcome to a world where freeze-dried delights become your allies in this noble quest.

**The role of diet in weight management**

Weight management is a multifaceted endeavor, and at its core, it hinges on one pivotal factor: diet. The food we consume plays an instrumental role in determining our weight, and more importantly, it significantly impacts our overall health and well-being.

Our dietary choices are intimately tied to our body weight. When we consume more calories than our bodies burn, the surplus energy is stored as fat, leading to weight gain. Conversely, when we eat fewer calories than we expend, we create a calorie deficit that results in weight loss. This fundamental principle is at the heart of any weight management strategy.

However, the simplicity of the "calories in, calories out" equation doesn't fully capture the complexity of a successful weight management plan. The quality and composition of the calories we consume matter just as much as the quantity. A diet rich in highly processed, calorie-dense foods, for instance, can lead to weight gain and a host of health problems, even if the calorie count remains low. Conversely, a diet centered around whole, nutrient-dense foods can support weight loss and foster optimal health.

Understanding the importance of diet in weight management is the first step towards achieving a healthier weight. It's not just about losing pounds; it's about adopting a sustainable, lifelong approach to eating that supports overall well-being. This is where freeze-dried foods come into play.

In the pages that follow, we'll explore how freeze-dried foods can help you make smarter dietary choices without sacrificing taste and nutrition. By harnessing the power of freeze-drying, we can create a bridge between our desire for convenient, delicious meals and our commitment to a healthier, more balanced lifestyle.

Get ready to embark on a journey of discovery, where you'll learn how freeze-dried delights can become your allies in the quest for effective weight management. The path to better health starts with your diet, and this book will equip you with the knowledge and tools to make informed choices, prioritize your health, and achieve your weight management goals.

**Introducing Freeze-Dried Foods as a Weight Loss Solution**

In the realm of weight management, the concept of a "magic bullet" solution is often met with skepticism, and for a good reason. Achieving and maintaining a healthy weight is a complex, individualized process that requires dedication, knowledge, and a sustainable approach. However, it's equally important to recognize that innovative and effective tools can greatly aid us in this journey.

Freeze-dried foods are one such tool. While they may not be a magical panacea for weight loss, they represent a powerful and often underestimated resource in our arsenal. These foods offer a unique combination of advantages that can make the path to weight management more achievable and enjoyable.

The process of freeze-drying involves preserving the taste, texture, and nutritional value of foods while removing their water content.

This technique results in lightweight, long-lasting, and nutrient-dense food items that are not only convenient but also versatile. Freeze-dried fruits, vegetables, proteins, and even beverages can be incorporated into your meals to support weight loss goals without compromising taste or nutrition.

As we journey through the chapters of this book, we will delve deeper into the science behind freeze-drying, explore the nutritional profile of freeze-dried foods, and provide practical guidance on how to integrate them into your daily diet. Whether you're seeking to manage your weight, curb cravings, or simply enjoy a more nutritious and flavorful diet, freeze-dried foods can play a pivotal role in your success.

This book is your comprehensive guide to understanding the potential of freeze-dried foods as a weight loss solution. We will equip you with the knowledge, strategies, and recipes needed to transform your relationship with food, make informed choices, and embark on a path toward better health. So, let's embark on this journey together, as we unlock the secrets of freeze-dried delights and explore how they can become a valuable ally in your quest for a healthier and happier you.

**Chapter 2: Understanding Freeze-Drying**

**Section 1: What is Freeze-Drying, and How Does It Work?**

Freeze-drying, often considered a form of culinary alchemy, is a meticulous process that transforms perishable foods into lightweight, shelf-stable delicacies while preserving their original taste, texture, and nutritional value. Understanding the intricate steps involved in freeze-drying can give you a deeper appreciation for this preservation technique.

**1. The Freeze-Drying Process:**

**Freezing:** The freeze-drying process begins by freezing the food to a very low temperature. This step locks in its freshness and prevents the growth of harmful microorganisms. The freezing phase is crucial because it sets the stage for moisture removal.

**Primary Drying:** After freezing, the food is placed in a vacuum chamber, where the temperature is gradually raised. This initiates a process known as sublimation, in which the frozen water within the food transitions directly from a solid (ice) to a gas (vapor) without passing through the liquid phase. This phase removes about 95% of the food's moisture content, effectively dehydrating it.

**Secondary Drying:** The secondary drying phase follows the primary drying, and its purpose is to remove the remaining moisture, typically around 5% or less. This stage involves a slightly higher temperature and helps ensure the food's long-term stability and shelf life. The secondary drying phase is critical for preventing the growth of spoilage microorganisms.

The entire process is controlled with precision, allowing food producers to maintain the integrity of the food. The result is a lightweight, crispy, and porous food product that's both delicious and nutritionally dense.

**2. Preservation of Nutrients and Flavor:**

Freeze-drying stands out as an exceptional method for preserving the nutritional content and flavor of foods. Unlike some other preservation methods that expose food to high heat, freeze-drying minimizes the degradation of sensitive vitamins, minerals, and enzymes. This means that the essential nutrients, such as vitamin C and fiber in fruits and vegetables, remain largely intact.

Furthermore, freeze-drying preserves the original taste and texture of foods. When you rehydrate a freeze-dried meal, you'll often find that it closely resembles the taste and mouthfeel of fresh food. This characteristic makes freeze-dried foods an attractive option for those who seek a balance between flavor and nutrition.

**3. Long Shelf Life:**

One of the remarkable benefits of freeze-dried foods is their extended shelf life. The removal of moisture during the freeze-drying process makes it difficult for microorganisms to grow and spoil the food. As a result, freeze-dried products can be stored for years, even decades, without the need for refrigeration or preservatives. This extended shelf life is not only convenient but also cost-effective, as it reduces food waste and allows you to keep a well-stocked pantry of nutritious options.

Understanding the intricacies of freeze-drying is key to appreciating its value in weight management and overall health. As you explore the following chapters, you'll see how these attributes of freeze-dried foods can work to your advantage, offering convenience, nutritional value, and a wide range of delicious options to support your weight loss journey.

**Section 2: Benefits of Freeze-Dried Foods for Weight Loss**

Freeze-dried foods provide a host of advantages that make them a valuable addition to your weight loss journey. In this section, we will delve into these benefits in more detail to help you understand why freeze-dried foods can be a powerful tool in achieving your weight management goals.

**1. Portion Control:**

Freeze-dried foods come in precisely measured portions, making it incredibly easy to control your calorie intake. Portion control is a critical aspect of weight management, as it helps you avoid overeating and stay within your daily caloric limits. With freeze-dried meals and snacks, you can have confidence in knowing exactly how much you're consuming, which is essential for maintaining a balanced diet and achieving your weight loss targets.

By having access to freeze-dried foods in controlled portion sizes, you can more effectively plan your meals and monitor your calorie intake, reducing the guesswork associated with traditional meal preparation.

**2. Low-Calorie Options:**

Many freeze-dried fruits and vegetables are naturally low in calories. This characteristic is particularly valuable for weight loss, as it allows you to indulge in satisfying, nutrient-rich snacks without exceeding your daily calorie budget. For example, a serving of freeze-dried strawberries or broccoli contains significantly fewer calories than their fresh counterparts.

These low-calorie options are excellent for filling the gap between meals, curbing cravings, and satisfying your hunger without compromising your weight loss goals. By incorporating freeze-dried foods into your daily routine, you can enjoy delicious, guilt-free snacks while working towards your target weight.

**3. Reduced Food Waste:**

Food waste is a significant concern in our modern society, both from an environmental and economic standpoint. Freeze-dried foods help combat this issue by having an exceptionally long shelf life. Unlike fresh produce, which can spoil quickly and lead to waste, freeze-dried items can be stored for extended periods without deterioration in quality or flavor.

The reduced food waste associated with freeze-dried foods means you're less likely to discard unused items, ultimately saving money and resources. This aligns with your weight loss objectives by promoting responsible consumption and supporting sustainability efforts.

By reducing food waste, freeze-dried foods also enable you to better manage portion sizes. You can prepare only the amount you need, avoiding leftovers that might tempt you to overindulge and hinder your progress towards a healthier weight.

The benefits of portion control, low-calorie options, and reduced food waste provided by freeze-dried foods can make a meaningful impact on your weight management efforts. As you continue to explore the possibilities of integrating these foods into your diet, you'll find that they not only support your goals but also offer convenience and satisfaction, making your weight loss journey more enjoyable and sustainable.

**Section 3: Common Misconceptions About Freeze-Dried Foods**

Misconceptions often swirl around new or less-familiar food preservation techniques, and freeze-drying is no exception. It's crucial to debunk these myths to make informed choices about incorporating freeze-dried foods into your weight loss journey.

**1. Myth: Freeze-Dried Foods Lack Nutritional Value:**

**Debunking the Myth:** This misconception couldn't be farther from the truth. Freeze-dried foods retain an impressive amount of their original nutritional value. The freeze-drying process involves minimal heat exposure, which helps preserve the sensitive vitamins and minerals in foods. As a result, freeze-dried fruits, vegetables, and proteins are often just as nutritious as their fresh counterparts.

In fact, freeze-dried foods can sometimes be even more nutritious because they are typically picked at the peak of ripeness, ensuring they are packed with essential nutrients. Additionally, since freeze-dried foods have a long shelf life, they allow you to consume nutrient-rich options all year round, regardless of the seasonal availability of fresh produce.

**2. Myth: Freeze-Dried Foods Are Expensive:**

**Debunking the Myth:** While it may seem that freeze-dried foods are a costly choice, they can actually be quite economical when you consider various factors. First, their extended shelf life significantly reduces food waste, which can save you money in the long run. You won't have to throw away spoiled groceries, and you can purchase freeze-dried items in bulk without the worry of spoilage.

Furthermore, the convenience of freeze-dried foods can lead to financial savings. For instance, you can reduce dining out expenses by having nutritious, easy-to-prepare freeze-dried meals on hand. They also eliminate the need for frequent grocery runs and offer greater control over portion sizes, reducing the temptation to overeat.

**3. Myth: Freeze-Dried Foods Lack Flavor:**

**Debunking the Myth:** Another common misconception is that freeze-dried foods lack flavor. In reality, freeze-dried foods are renowned for retaining the natural taste and aroma of fresh ingredients. The freeze-drying process preserves the volatile compounds responsible for flavor, resulting in foods that closely mimic their fresh counterparts when rehydrated.

The diversity of freeze-dried options available, from fruits and vegetables to meats and even desserts, allows you to create a wide range of flavorful dishes. When prepared thoughtfully, freeze-dried ingredients can elevate your meals and snacks with their delicious and authentic taste.

By dispelling these misconceptions, you can gain a more accurate understanding of freeze-dried foods and their role in your weight loss journey. The reality is that freeze-dried foods offer a host of benefits, including exceptional nutrition, cost-effectiveness, and a taste that's hard to beat. As you explore the upcoming chapters, you'll have the confidence to embrace freeze-dried foods as a valuable component of your balanced and healthy diet.

Chapter 3: Freeze-Dried Foods and Nutritional Value

**Section 1: Comparing the Nutritional Content of Fresh, Frozen, and Freeze-Dried Foods**

To truly appreciate the nutritional value of freeze-dried foods, it's essential to compare them to their fresh and frozen counterparts. This section provides an in-depth examination of how freeze-dried foods stack up against fresh and frozen options in terms of nutritional content.

**Fresh Foods:**

Fresh fruits, vegetables, and proteins are often considered the gold standard for nutrition. When harvested at their peak of ripeness, they offer a burst of flavor and a rich array of vitamins, minerals, and antioxidants. However, the nutritional value of fresh foods begins to decline as soon as they are harvested due to exposure to air, light, and temperature variations.

The journey from the farm to your plate can take time, leading to potential nutrient degradation during transportation and storage. This means that even if you're diligent about buying fresh, locally-sourced produce, you might not be getting the full spectrum of nutrients you expect.

**Frozen Foods:**

Freezing is an effective method for preserving the nutritional value of foods. When foods are frozen shortly after harvest or processing, they lock in their nutrients, and this preservation can be maintained throughout storage.

However, it's essential to recognize that freezing is not without its consequences. While it does a great job of preserving many nutrients, some water-soluble vitamins (like vitamin C) can be sensitive to freezing temperatures. When foods are frozen, some of these vitamins can leach into the ice crystals that form, potentially reducing the overall nutrient content.

**Comparing Nutrient Retention:**

Scientific studies have shown that freeze-dried foods can retain a remarkable portion of their original nutrients. This is primarily due to the unique freeze-drying process. Freeze-drying involves freezing the food and then slowly reducing the surrounding pressure, allowing the frozen water within the food to sublimate, or transform directly from ice to vapor, without passing through a liquid phase.

This method preserves the structural integrity of the food and minimizes nutrient loss. For example, research has demonstrated that freeze-dried fruits and vegetables can retain the majority of their vitamin and mineral content, as well as important antioxidants. This means that you can enjoy the benefits of these nutrients without worrying about significant losses.

In summary, freeze-dried foods offer a compelling advantage when it comes to preserving the nutritional content of foods. While fresh and frozen foods are valuable components of a healthy diet, freeze-dried options can complement them by providing a nutrient-rich, convenient, and shelf-stable alternative that contributes to your overall nutrition and supports your weight management goals.

**Section 2: How Freeze-Drying Preserves Essential Nutrients**

Freeze-drying, also known as lyophilization, is an exceptional food preservation method renowned for its ability to maintain the essential nutrients in foods. In this section, we'll delve into the science behind freeze-drying and how it effectively preserves the nutritional value of foods.

**Minimal Heat Exposure:**

One of the primary reasons freeze-drying is so effective at nutrient preservation is its minimal heat exposure. Unlike traditional preservation methods like canning or pasteurization, which subject foods to high temperatures, freeze-drying utilizes cold temperatures for a significant portion of the process.

The freeze-drying process begins with freezing the food, which helps to lock in its original nutrients. The food is then placed in a vacuum chamber, and the temperature is gradually raised. This initiates a process known as sublimation, in which the frozen water within the food transitions directly from a solid (ice) to a gas (vapor) without passing through the liquid phase. Because the food remains frozen during the sublimation phase, minimal heat is applied, preventing the breakdown of sensitive vitamins and other heat-sensitive compounds.

**Volatile Compounds Preservation:**

One remarkable aspect of freeze-drying is its ability to preserve the volatile compounds responsible for the flavors and aromas of foods. Many of the compounds that contribute to the delicious taste and smell of foods are highly sensitive to heat. Conventional drying methods often lead to the loss of these compounds, resulting in a less flavorful end product.

Freeze-drying, with its gentle temperature control, preserves these volatile compounds, making freeze-dried foods closely resemble their fresh counterparts when rehydrated. For instance, freeze-dried strawberries retain their sweet, vibrant flavor, and herbs maintain their aromatic qualities, allowing you to enjoy the natural taste and scent of these ingredients in your meals and snacks.

**Retention of Fiber:**

Dietary fiber is a critical component of a healthy diet, aiding in digestion and promoting a feeling of fullness. Many fresh and frozen fruits and vegetables are excellent sources of fiber. When foods are subjected to traditional drying or canning processes, their fiber content can be compromised.

Freeze-drying, with its minimal heat exposure, helps retain the dietary fiber present in the original foods. This is important for weight management because high-fiber foods can help control appetite and support your efforts to maintain or lose weight. Including freeze-dried fruits and vegetables in your diet allows you to benefit from their fiber content without sacrificing their taste or texture.

In summary, freeze-drying is a preservation method that excels in retaining the essential nutrients, flavors, and aromas of foods. By minimizing heat exposure and preserving volatile compounds and fiber, freeze-dried foods provide you with a nutritious, delicious, and convenient option for supporting your weight management and overall health goals.

**Section 3: The Role of Freeze-Dried Fruits, Vegetables, and Proteins in a Balanced Diet**

Freeze-dried foods, including fruits, vegetables, and proteins, can play a significant role in helping you achieve a balanced and healthy diet. In this section, we will explore how each of these freeze-dried categories contributes to a well-rounded and nutritionally sound eating plan.

**Fruits:**

Freeze-dried fruits are a flavorful and nutritious addition to your diet. Here's how they can enhance your nutritional intake and weight management efforts:

1. **Convenience:** Freeze-dried fruits offer the convenience of fresh fruit without the need for refrigeration. They are lightweight and shelf-stable, making them an excellent choice for on-the-go snacking. This convenience ensures that you have access to nutrient-rich options wherever you are, helping you resist less healthy snack choices.

2. **Vitamins and Antioxidants:** Freeze-dried fruits retain their original vitamins and antioxidants. They provide essential nutrients like vitamin C, which supports the immune system, and antioxidants that combat oxidative stress in the body. These nutrients are integral to overall health and well-being.

3. **Satisfying Sweet Cravings:** Freeze-dried fruits can be a satisfying alternative to sugary snacks. They offer natural sweetness and a satisfying crunch, helping you curb your sweet tooth while avoiding excessive added sugars, which can contribute to weight gain.

4. **Dietary Fiber:** Many fruits are high in dietary fiber, which aids in digestion and provides a feeling of fullness. High-fiber snacks can help you control your appetite, making freeze-dried fruits a valuable addition to your weight management plan.

**Vegetables:**

Freeze-dried vegetables are versatile and nutritious. Here's how they contribute to a balanced diet:

1. **Nutrient Density:** Freeze-dried vegetables are nutrient-dense, providing essential vitamins and minerals like vitamin K, folate, and potassium. These nutrients support various bodily functions, from bone health to heart function.

2. **Dietary Fiber:** Vegetables are often excellent sources of dietary fiber, which promotes digestion and helps maintain healthy cholesterol levels. Including freeze-dried vegetables in your diet ensures you benefit from their fiber content without the hassle of cooking and preparation.

3. **Sustainability:** Freeze-dried vegetables are lightweight and have a long shelf life, reducing food waste. They allow you to consume a variety of vegetables year-round, supporting your health and sustainability goals.

4. **Flavorful Cooking:** Freeze-dried vegetables can enhance the flavors of your cooked meals. They add a burst of taste to soups, stir-fries, and pasta dishes, making it easier to enjoy a balanced and nutritious diet.

**Proteins:**

Freeze-dried proteins, whether they are lean meats or plant-based alternatives, are valuable sources of essential amino acids and play a vital role in a balanced diet:

1. **Muscle Maintenance and Growth:** Proteins are the building blocks of muscle and are essential for maintaining and building lean body mass. Including freeze-dried proteins in your meals ensures you get the amino acids needed to support your muscles, which is particularly important for active individuals.

2. **Satiety:** Protein-rich foods help you feel full and satisfied, reducing the likelihood of overeating and snacking on less nutritious options. This satiety can support your weight management goals by curbing hunger.

3. **Convenience:** Freeze-dried proteins are easy to incorporate into your meals. They rehydrate quickly and are suitable for various recipes, making it convenient to add protein to your diet without extensive meal preparation.

By incorporating freeze-dried fruits, vegetables, and proteins into your daily meals and snacks, you can enjoy the convenience, nutrition, and versatility they offer. These freeze-dried options help you maintain a well-rounded diet, which is vital for weight management, overall health, and long-term well-being.

Chapter 4: Meal Planning with Freeze-Dried Foods

**Section 1: How to Incorporate Freeze-Dried Foods into Your Daily Meals**

Incorporating freeze-dried foods into your daily meals is a practical and flavorful way to elevate your diet. This section will guide you through various mealtime opportunities, highlighting how freeze-dried foods can be seamlessly integrated into your breakfast, lunch, dinner, and snack routines.

**Breakfast:**

1. *Cereals and Oatmeal:* Start your day with a burst of fruity flavor and nutrition by adding freeze-dried berries, mango, or bananas to your cereal or oatmeal. These fruits not only provide essential vitamins and antioxidants but also create a delightful crunch that adds a new dimension to your breakfast.

2. *Yogurt Parfaits:* Layer freeze-dried fruits like strawberries, blueberries, or peaches with yogurt and granola to create a satisfying and visually appealing breakfast parfait. The fruits' natural sweetness and tartness pair wonderfully with the creaminess of yogurt.

3. *Smoothies:* Blend freeze-dried fruits into your morning smoothies for a convenient and nutritious boost. Whether you prefer a classic strawberry-banana blend or a tropical pineapple-mango concoction, freeze-dried fruits add flavor and vitamins without the hassle of fresh fruit preparation.

**Lunch:**

1. *Salads:* Freeze-dried vegetables make it easy to elevate your salads. Add a handful of freeze-dried corn, peas, or bell peppers to create a burst of color, texture, and nutrition. These vegetables rehydrate quickly, making them a hassle-free addition to your salad.

2. *Sandwiches and Wraps:* Include freeze-dried vegetables like spinach or kale for a fresh, crispy crunch in your sandwiches and wraps. They not only provide a unique texture but also an extra layer of nutrients.

3. *Soups:** Freeze-dried vegetables are excellent for soups. Whether it's a classic chicken noodle soup with freeze-dried carrots and peas or a hearty vegetable soup, these ingredients enhance the flavor and nutrition of your soup without the need for extensive chopping and prep work.

**Dinner:**

1. *Stir-Fries:* Freeze-dried proteins, whether chicken, beef, or tofu, can be rehydrated and used in stir-fry dishes. Their lightweight and shelf-stable nature make them an excellent choice for creating

quick and satisfying meals. Pair them with freeze-dried vegetables and your favorite stir-fry sauce for a delicious and balanced dinner.

2. *Pasta Dishes:* Freeze-dried proteins can also be incorporated into pasta dishes. Add rehydrated shrimp to your seafood linguine or mix in freeze-dried chicken with fettuccine alfredo for a simple yet flavorful dinner option.

**Snacks:**

1. *Snack Mixes:** Create your own nutritious snack mixes by combining freeze-dried fruits and nuts. For example, a mix of freeze-dried apples, almonds, and dried cranberries offers a balanced blend of flavors and textures, perfect for on-the-go snacking.

2. *Trail Mix:** Customize your trail mix with freeze-dried fruits, such as strawberries or pineapple, for a sweet and tangy twist. Pair them with nuts, seeds, and dark chocolate chips for a satisfying and energy-boosting snack.

3. *Flavored Popcorn:** Sprinkle freeze-dried fruit powders, like raspberry or blueberry, on freshly popped popcorn for a unique and healthy twist. These powders provide natural flavors without the added sugars or artificial ingredients often found in store-bought popcorn seasonings.

Incorporating freeze-dried foods into your daily meals is a versatile and time-saving way to enhance your diet. Their convenience, long shelf life, and rich nutrient content make them a valuable addition to your culinary endeavors, ensuring that you enjoy both the flavor and health benefits of these foods with ease.

**Section 2: Creating a Well-Balanced Freeze-Dried Food Pantry**

Building a well-balanced freeze-dried food pantry is an essential aspect of making the most of these versatile, nutritious ingredients. This section offers guidance on stocking and maintaining a pantry that supports your dietary needs and goals.

**Diversity:**

1. **Fruits:** Ensure that your pantry includes a diverse selection of freeze-dried fruits. You can choose from options like strawberries, blueberries, apples, mangoes, and bananas. Different fruits offer various vitamins, minerals, and antioxidants. A variety of freeze-dried fruits allows you to enjoy a wide range of flavors and nutrients in your meals and snacks.

2. **Vegetables:** Stock up on a variety of freeze-dried vegetables, such as peas, corn, bell peppers, kale, and spinach. Including an assortment of vegetables ensures that you have options for salads, soups, sandwiches, and more. Each vegetable brings unique nutrients and flavors to your dishes.

3. **Proteins:** Freeze-dried proteins can include options like chicken, beef, shrimp, or plant-based alternatives like tofu. Having a mix of these proteins provides versatility in meal preparation, catering to different dietary preferences and needs.

**Shelf Life and Storage:**

1. **Optimal Storage Conditions:** To maintain the long shelf life of freeze-dried foods, store them in a cool, dry, and dark place. This prevents exposure to heat, moisture, and light, which can degrade the quality of these foods over time. Proper storage ensures that your freeze-dried foods remain fresh and nutritious for extended periods.

2. **Sealable Containers:** Consider using airtight, sealable containers or Mylar bags for packaging freeze-dried foods. This

helps protect them from moisture, pests, and oxygen, which can compromise their shelf life and quality.

3. **Labeling:** Labeling your freeze-dried foods with the date of purchase can be helpful for rotation. Ensuring that older items are used first prevents waste and guarantees that your pantry remains well-stocked with fresh ingredients.

**Inventory Management:**

1. **Rotation:** Practicing a first-in, first-out (FIFO) rotation system ensures that you consume freeze-dried foods before they reach their expiration dates. As you purchase new items, place them at the back of your pantry and use older items from the front. This strategy minimizes waste and keeps your pantry efficiently stocked.

2. **Regular Assessment:** Periodically assess your freeze-dried food inventory to identify items that need to be used or rotated. This process can help you plan your meals around items that may have a shorter shelf life.

By following these guidelines, you'll create a well-organized and balanced freeze-dried food pantry that not only supports your dietary needs but also contributes to a sustainable and cost-effective approach to meal planning. A well-stocked and well-maintained pantry enables you to prepare nutritious, convenient, and flavorful meals with ease.

**Section 3: Sample Meal Plans and Recipes**

This section provides practical meal plans and recipes, demonstrating how you can make the most of freeze-dried foods in your daily meals. Whether it's breakfast, lunch, dinner, or snacks, the following ideas showcase the convenience and versatility of incorporating freeze-dried ingredients into your diet:

**Breakfast:**

1. *Fruit-Filled Oatmeal:* Start your day with a hearty bowl of oatmeal. Top it with rehydrated freeze-dried strawberries, blueberries, or raspberries for a burst of flavor and nutrition. Add a drizzle of honey or a dollop of Greek yogurt for extra creaminess.

2. *Tropical Smoothie:* Blend freeze-dried mango, pineapple, and banana with yogurt and a splash of coconut milk for a refreshing tropical smoothie. The natural sweetness and vibrant colors of these fruits make your morning routine even more enjoyable.

3. *Berry Parfait:** Create a yogurt parfait by layering freeze-dried blueberries, granola, and your favorite yogurt. This combination offers a delightful mix of textures and flavors, along with the nutritional benefits of yogurt and berries.

**Lunch:**

1. *Garden Salad:** Prepare a fresh garden salad with mixed greens, cherry tomatoes, and cucumbers. Top it off with freeze-dried bell peppers, peas, and corn for added crunch and a pop of color. Drizzle your favorite dressing for a satisfying lunch option.

2. *Veggie Wrap:* Construct a veggie wrap using whole-grain tortillas, hummus, and a blend of freeze-dried vegetables such as kale, spinach, and bell peppers. The crunchy, rehydrated veggies pair perfectly with creamy hummus.

3. *Tomato Basil Soup:** Enjoy a classic tomato basil soup by rehydrating freeze-dried tomatoes and basil in vegetable or chicken broth. This comforting and nutritious soup can be made in minutes.

**Dinner:**

1. *Chicken Stir-Fry:** Prepare a quick and tasty chicken stir-fry by rehydrating freeze-dried chicken and adding it to a pan with stir-fried vegetables. You can include a mix of freeze-dried bell peppers, broccoli, and carrots for a colorful and satisfying dish. Serve it over brown rice or noodles with your choice of sauce.

2. *Beef Stroganoff:** Make a savory beef stroganoff by rehydrating freeze-dried beef and serving it in a creamy mushroom sauce. Pair it with egg noodles or rice for a hearty, homemade meal.

3. *Pasta Primavera:** Create a pasta primavera using freeze-dried bell peppers, zucchini, and peas. Toss these rehydrated veggies with cooked pasta and a light olive oil and herb dressing for a fresh and vibrant dinner option.

**Snacks:**

1. *Nutty Fruit Mix:** Make a nutritious snack mix by combining freeze-dried fruits like strawberries and blueberries with nuts, such as almonds and cashews. This blend offers a perfect balance of sweetness and crunch for your midday pick-me-up.

2. *Tropical Trail Mix:** Craft a tropical-inspired trail mix by mixing freeze-dried pineapple, coconut flakes, and macadamia nuts. This exotic combination provides a unique and satisfying snack for your outdoor adventures.

3. *Fruity Popcorn:** Sprinkle freeze-dried fruit powders, such as raspberry or blueberry, on freshly popped popcorn. This DIY popcorn seasoning adds a delightful fruity twist to your movie night or afternoon snacking.

These sample meal plans and recipes illustrate the creativity and convenience that freeze-dried foods can bring to your meals and snacks. They offer endless possibilities for elevating your daily diet with the natural flavors, nutrition, and extended shelf life of freeze-dried ingredients.


Chapter 5: Freeze-Dried Foods and Weight Loss

**Section 1: Benefits of Freeze-Dried Foods for Weight Loss**

Freeze-dried foods offer several advantages that can significantly contribute to your weight loss journey. Understanding these benefits can empower you to make informed dietary choices and leverage freeze-dried foods to achieve your weight management goals.

**1. Nutrient Density:**

Freeze-dried foods are nutrient powerhouses. They retain the majority of their original vitamins, minerals, and antioxidants during the freeze-drying process. This means that even in their lightweight, shelf-stable form, freeze-dried foods can provide essential nutrients crucial for your overall health. When you're focusing on weight loss, it's essential to consume nutrient-dense foods to meet your body's requirements while keeping your calorie intake in check. Freeze-dried fruits and vegetables can help you achieve this balance by offering substantial nutrition without excessive calories.

**2. Low-Calorie Options:**

Many freeze-dried fruits and vegetables are naturally low in calories. Since water content is removed during the freeze-drying process, the resulting product is calorie-dense, meaning you get more nutrients per calorie. For instance, a serving of freeze-dried fruit may be much smaller in volume than its fresh counterpart, but it contains a comparable amount of essential vitamins and minerals. This makes freeze-dried foods an excellent choice for those who want to feel full and satisfied without consuming excessive calories.

The fiber in these foods can also promote satiety, helping you control your appetite.

**3. Portion Control:**

Effective portion control is a key strategy in weight management. Freeze-dried foods are pre-portioned, often coming in single-serving packages. This eliminates the guesswork when it comes to portion sizes and helps you avoid overindulging. Whether you're packing a snack for work or including freeze-dried ingredients in your meal planning, you can rely on the convenience of portion-controlled options to stay on track with your calorie goals.

**4. Long Shelf Life:**

The extended shelf life of freeze-dried foods is another advantage for weight loss. It reduces the likelihood of food waste and helps you maintain a consistent supply of healthy options. Knowing you have nutritious freeze-dried foods readily available discourages impulsive decisions to opt for less healthy, calorie-dense alternatives when you're hungry and in a hurry. This convenience can be a game-changer when trying to stick to your weight loss plan.

**5. Convenience:**

Freeze-dried foods offer exceptional convenience. Whether you're at home, work, or on the go, they can be easily integrated into your diet. They require no refrigeration or preparation, making them the perfect choice for a quick, healthy snack. This convenience ensures you always have a nutritious option available, reducing the temptation to grab calorie-laden, less healthy alternatives when you're pressed for time.

In summary, freeze-dried foods are a valuable asset for weight loss. Their nutrient density, low-calorie content, portion control, long shelf life, and convenience make them an ideal choice for those seeking to achieve and maintain a healthy weight. By incorporating freeze-dried foods into your diet, you can enjoy flavorful, satisfying meals and snacks that support your weight management goals effectively.

**Section 2: Strategies for Portion Control**

Portion control is a critical aspect of managing your weight effectively. It ensures that you consume the right amount of calories to support your goals without overindulging. Freeze-dried foods can be an essential tool in achieving portion control, whether you're planning your meals or simply grabbing a quick snack. Here are strategies to help you manage your portions:

**1. Pre-Portioned Snacks:**

One of the most convenient aspects of freeze-dried foods is that they often come in pre-portioned, single-serving packages. This pre-packaging eliminates the need for measuring or guessing portion sizes. Whether you're reaching for a snack at work or packing something for a hike, you can rely on these portion-controlled options to help you stay on track with your calorie goals.

**2. Meal Preparation:**

Integrating freeze-dried foods into your meal planning enables precise portion control. You can easily calculate the number of servings you need and prepare dishes with consistent portion sizes. For example, if you're making a stir-fry, rehydrate a specific amount of freeze-dried vegetables to ensure you include the right portion in your meal. This practice helps you manage your calorie intake accurately while enjoying nutritious and flavorful meals.

**3. Tracking Intake:**

Keeping a record of your daily food intake can help you stay mindful of your portion sizes and calorie consumption. Freeze-dried foods simplify the tracking process because they typically come in clearly marked, portion-controlled packaging. By recording the freeze-dried items you consume, you can easily calculate their nutritional content and monitor your calorie intake. There are various mobile apps and online tools that can assist you in this process, making it more manageable and helping you stay on course with your weight loss goals.

**4. Mindful Eating:**

Practice mindful eating to become more attuned to your body's hunger and fullness cues. Eating slowly, savoring each bite, and paying attention to the flavors and textures of your meals can help you recognize when you're satisfied. Freeze-dried foods can be an excellent aid in this practice because they provide a concentrated burst of flavor and nutrition. Taking the time to appreciate the taste of freeze-dried fruits or vegetables can help you feel more satisfied with smaller portions.

**5. Measuring Tools:**

Use measuring tools, such as cups, spoons, or a food scale, to measure freeze-dried ingredients when preparing meals. This ensures accuracy in portion control and helps you meet your dietary objectives. For instance, if you're adding freeze-dried fruit to your yogurt, measuring it out will help you maintain the desired portion size and calorie count.

By incorporating these portion control strategies into your daily routine and making the most of freeze-dried foods, you can effectively manage your calorie intake and support your weight loss goals. Portion control not only aids in weight loss but also encourages a healthier and more balanced approach to eating, which is crucial for long-term success in managing your weight.

**Section 3: Meal Planning Techniques for Weight Loss**

Effective meal planning is a key aspect of successful weight management. With the convenience, nutrition, and long shelf life of freeze-dried foods, you can streamline your meal planning and make it more conducive to your weight loss goals. Here are meal planning techniques that leverage freeze-dried foods:

**1. Balanced Meals:**

Incorporate a variety of freeze-dried fruits, vegetables, and proteins into your meals to create balanced dishes that provide essential nutrients while managing your calorie intake. Consider the following strategies:

- **Fruits for Breakfast:** Start your day with a serving of freeze-dried fruits. Sprinkle them on your cereal or oatmeal, mix them into yogurt, or blend them into a smoothie. These options add flavor and nutrition to your breakfast while promoting a sense of fullness.

- **Vegetables for Lunch:** Freeze-dried vegetables can enhance your lunchtime salads, sandwiches, or wraps. They add color, texture, and essential nutrients to your midday meals without the need for extensive prep work.

- **Proteins for Dinner:** Incorporate freeze-dried proteins, such as chicken, beef, or plant-based alternatives, into your dinner recipes. They are lightweight and easy to rehydrate, making them convenient for stir-fries, pasta dishes, and other main courses.

**2. Snacking:**

Plan for healthy freeze-dried snacks to prevent impulsive choices that may not align with your weight loss goals. Having a selection of portion-controlled, nutritious snacks readily available can help curb cravings and reduce your calorie consumption. Here are some snacking strategies:

- **Pre-Packaged Snacks:** Take advantage of pre-packaged freeze-dried snacks, like fruit crisps or vegetable chips. Their single-serving portions make it easy to satisfy your snack cravings without overindulging.

- **DIY Snack Mixes:** Create your own nutritious snack mixes using a variety of freeze-dried ingredients. Combine freeze-dried fruits, nuts, and seeds to create a balanced and satisfying snack blend. Experiment with different flavor combinations to keep your snacking exciting and in line with your weight loss goals.

- **Trail Mix:** Customize your trail mix with freeze-dried fruits, nuts, seeds, and dark chocolate chips for a satisfying and energy-boosting snack. The variety of textures and flavors makes this option ideal for a quick pick-me-up.

**3. Calorie Control:**

Freeze-dried foods are naturally portioned and are often lower in calories than many processed snacks. By including them in your meal plans, you can control your calorie intake more effectively. Here are techniques for calorie control:

- **Calorie Counting:** Use nutritional information labels provided on freeze-dried food packaging to monitor your calorie intake. This practice ensures that you stay within your desired calorie range.

- **Meal Prepping:** Plan and prepare your meals in advance using freeze-dried ingredients. This gives you more control over the number of calories in your meals and allows you to meet your specific dietary goals.

- **Nutrient-Rich Choices:** Select freeze-dried foods that are rich in essential nutrients and lower in calories. Fruits and vegetables are often excellent choices because they offer vitamins, minerals, and fiber with fewer calories compared to some other snack options.

**4. Versatility:**

Freeze-dried foods are versatile ingredients that can be used in various recipes. Here are some ways to incorporate freeze-dried foods into your meals:

- **Soups:** Add freeze-dried vegetables to your homemade soups to increase their nutritional value and flavor. Rehydrate the vegetables in broth or water before adding them to your soup pot.

- **Stir-Fries:** Freeze-dried proteins, such as chicken or beef, can be rehydrated and incorporated into stir-fry dishes. Pair them with freeze-dried vegetables and your favorite stir-fry sauce for a quick and flavorful meal.

- **Salads:** Enhance your salads with freeze-dried vegetables, which offer a satisfying crunch and a burst of flavor. Simply rehydrate the vegetables and mix them into your favorite salad greens.

- **Snacks:** Incorporate freeze-dried fruits and vegetables into your snack recipes. For example, you can create delicious fruit and nut bars with freeze-dried berries or add freeze-dried vegetables to homemade kale chips for a crunchy and nutritious snack.

By making use of these meal planning techniques, you can harness the benefits of freeze-dried foods to streamline your weight loss journey. These techniques not only aid in controlling your calorie intake but also enable you to maintain a well-balanced and nutrient-dense diet that supports your overall health and wellness.

Chapter 6: Staying Motivated and Overcoming Challenges

**Section 1: Staying Motivated**

Staying motivated throughout your weight loss journey is a fundamental component of long-term success. Here, we delve into strategies to keep you inspired and on track, ensuring that your motivation remains high even when faced with challenges:

**1. Set Clear Goals:**

Establishing specific, measurable, and achievable goals is the first step in maintaining motivation. Whether it's a target weight, a fitness achievement, or a clothing size, having a clear goal provides you with a tangible endpoint to work towards. Break down your larger goal into smaller, manageable milestones. These smaller victories can provide a continuous sense of accomplishment and motivation.

**2. Visualize Your Success:**

Visualization is a powerful tool for staying motivated. Create a vivid mental image of yourself after achieving your weight loss goals. Imagine the way you'll look, feel, and the positive changes in your life. Visualizing success makes your goals more concrete and helps you stay committed.

**3. Track Your Progress:**

Keeping a record of your achievements is crucial for maintaining motivation. Maintain a food diary, fitness journal, or use a mobile app to track your progress. Recording your daily exercise routines, meals, and even your emotional states can offer insights into your habits and help you see how far you've come. It's an excellent way to remind yourself of your dedication and the results you've achieved.

**4. Reward Yourself:**

Rewarding yourself for meeting your milestones is a powerful motivator. Set up a system of rewards for achieving your goals, whether they are big or small. These rewards don't need to be extravagant; they can be as simple as treating yourself to a favorite book, a spa day, or a relaxing evening at home. Recognizing your efforts with a reward provides positive reinforcement for your accomplishments.

**5. Find a Support System:**

Connecting with friends, family, or a support group can be invaluable for maintaining motivation. Sharing your journey with others who understand your struggles and successes can be an incredible source of encouragement. Support groups, whether in-person or online, provide a community of like-minded individuals who can offer advice, motivation, and accountability.

**6. Stay Informed:**

Educating yourself about the benefits of a healthy lifestyle, including the positive impact on your physical and mental well-being, can help maintain motivation. Understanding the science behind weight loss, the importance of a balanced diet, and the role of exercise can reinforce the significance of your journey. Learning about the long-term benefits can provide a solid foundation for your motivation.

By applying these strategies for staying motivated, you can bolster your determination and focus, ensuring that you remain committed to your weight loss goals. Remember that motivation can fluctuate, but with the right tools and support, you can navigate the challenges and continue moving forward.

**Section 2: Overcoming Challenges**

Weight loss journeys come with their fair share of challenges. Recognizing and addressing these obstacles is vital for maintaining progress and staying motivated. Here are strategies to overcome common challenges:

**1. Plateaus:**

Weight loss plateaus are normal and can be disheartening. When you reach a plateau, it's essential to remember that it's part of the process. To overcome plateaus, consider:

- **Changing Your Exercise Routine:** Alter your workout regimen by trying different exercises, increasing the intensity, or introducing new activities. This change can shock your body out of a plateau.

- **Reassessing Your Diet:** Review your dietary habits and portion sizes. Sometimes, minor adjustments, such as reducing portion sizes or limiting certain foods, can help break through a plateau.

- **Seeking Professional Guidance:** If you're consistently struggling with plateaus, consider consulting a healthcare professional, nutritionist, or personal trainer for personalized advice and strategies to overcome them.

**2. Emotional Eating:**

Emotional eating is a common challenge in weight loss. It often involves turning to food for comfort during stressful or emotional moments. Strategies to overcome emotional eating include:

- **Identifying Triggers:** Recognize the emotional triggers that lead to overeating. Common triggers include stress, boredom, sadness, or anxiety. Once you identify these triggers, you can work on alternative coping mechanisms.

- **Healthy Coping Strategies:** Replace emotional eating with healthier coping strategies, such as exercise, meditation, journaling, or talking to a friend. These alternatives can provide emotional relief without the negative consequences of overeating.

**3. Cravings:**

Cravings for certain foods can be strong and challenging to resist. To manage cravings, consider the following:

- **Healthy Substitutes:** Keep healthy, low-calorie alternatives on hand to satisfy your cravings. For example, if you're craving something sweet, reach for a piece of fruit or a small serving of dark chocolate.

- **Meal Planning:** Plan your meals and snacks ahead of time. Having a structured meal plan can help reduce the intensity of cravings and prevent impulsive, unhealthy choices.

**4. Social Pressure:**

Social gatherings and peer pressure can make it challenging to stick to your dietary and exercise plans. Strategies for dealing with social pressure include:

- **Communication:** Inform your friends and family about your weight loss goals. When they understand your objectives, they can offer support by suggesting healthier dining options or respecting your dietary choices when hosting events.

- **Make Healthy Choices:** When dining out or attending social events, look for healthier menu options. Many restaurants offer nutritious choices that align with your weight loss goals.

**5. Time Management:**

Balancing work, family, and your weight loss journey can be demanding. Effective time management and planning are key to overcoming this challenge. Strategies include:

- **Prioritizing Health:** Make your health a top priority. Schedule regular workouts, meal planning, and grocery shopping into your day to ensure you maintain a consistent routine.

- **Efficiency:** Look for ways to make your fitness and meal preparation more efficient. Short, high-intensity workouts and batch cooking are examples of time-saving strategies.

**6. Self-Criticism:**

It's easy to become your harshest critic, especially when the scale doesn't show the results you desire. To overcome self-criticism:

- **Practice Self-Compassion:** Be kind to yourself and practice self-compassion. Understand that progress is rarely linear, and setbacks are part of the journey. Celebrate your achievements and don't be too hard on yourself during challenging moments.

By applying these strategies for overcoming common weight loss challenges, you can navigate potential obstacles with greater ease and resilience. Remember that setbacks are a normal part of the journey, and with the right mindset and support, you can continue progressing towards your goals.

**Section 3: Long-Term Sustainability**

Long-term sustainability is the ultimate objective of your weight loss journey. It's about adopting lasting, healthier habits that allow you to maintain your weight, fitness, and overall well-being. Here are strategies to ensure that your progress is not only temporary but sustainable for the years to come:

**1. Gradual Changes:**

Sustainability begins with the gradual integration of new, healthier habits into your lifestyle. Avoid radical, unsustainable diets or exercise regimens. Instead, focus on making small, consistent changes that are easier to maintain over time. These might include gradually reducing portion sizes, incorporating more fruits and vegetables into your meals, or increasing your physical activity in manageable increments.

**2. Consistency:**

Consistency is paramount for long-term sustainability. Continue to engage in the healthy habits that helped you achieve your weight loss goals. Consistency should apply to both your dietary choices and your exercise routine. Regular, balanced meals and workouts become ingrained behaviors that are less likely to be abandoned.

**3. Variety:**

Variety in your diet and exercise routine helps maintain interest and motivation. Over time, your taste preferences and workout interests may evolve. Embrace this by trying new foods, recipes, or exercises. A diverse diet ensures you receive a wide range of nutrients, and changing up your workouts can prevent monotony and plateaus.

**4. Mindful Eating:**

Practice mindful eating as a long-term strategy. Mindful eating involves savoring each bite, paying attention to hunger and fullness cues, and enjoying your food without distractions. This approach promotes a healthier relationship with food, helping to prevent overeating and mindless snacking. As a sustainable practice, it encourages a positive and balanced approach to eating.

**5. Seek Professional Guidance:**

Consult a registered dietitian or nutritionist to develop a sustainable meal plan tailored to your specific needs. Regular check-ins with a healthcare professional can help you stay accountable and address any challenges that arise. These professionals can provide ongoing guidance, adapt your dietary plan as your needs change, and help you navigate any nutrition-related obstacles.

**6. Stay Active:**

Maintaining an active lifestyle is crucial for long-term sustainability. Regular exercise not only supports weight maintenance but also contributes to your overall well-being. Incorporate physical activities you enjoy into your daily routine, whether it's jogging, swimming, yoga, or dancing. The key is to make exercise a natural and enjoyable part of your life.

**7. Keep Setting Goals:**

While your initial weight loss goal may have been met, setting new goals is a way to maintain motivation and focus on continued improvement. These goals can involve improving fitness, trying new physical challenges, or simply maintaining your current weight. By setting goals, you provide yourself with ongoing motivation and direction.

**8. Build a Supportive Environment:**

Surround yourself with a supportive environment that encourages healthy choices. If possible, create a home environment that is conducive to your goals, and establish routines that align with your healthier lifestyle. Maintain a support network of friends and family who understand and respect your choices.

**9. Stay Educated:**

Continuously educate yourself about nutrition, exercise, and health. The more you understand about these topics, the better equipped you are to make informed choices and maintain your healthy habits. Stay updated on the latest research and trends in health and wellness to ensure your approach remains relevant and effective.

By following these strategies for long-term sustainability, you can transform your weight loss journey into a sustainable and fulfilling lifestyle. The ultimate goal is not only to achieve a target weight but also to lead a healthier, happier life while maintaining your well-being for the years to come.

Chapter 7: Freeze-Dried Foods and the Future of Weight Management

**Section 1: Advancements in Freeze-Dried Foods**

The freeze-drying process has seen significant advancements, transforming freeze-dried foods into a viable solution for weight management and overall well-being. These advancements are poised to shape the future of freeze-dried foods and their role in healthy living. Here's a closer look at some of the notable advancements:

**1. Enhanced Nutrition:**

Advancements in freeze-drying techniques have focused on retaining as many of the original nutrients in foods as possible. Traditional drying methods often result in significant nutrient loss due to exposure to high heat. Freeze-drying, with its gentle process of freezing and sublimation, helps preserve the natural vitamins, minerals, and antioxidants in foods. Ongoing research seeks to improve this preservation even further.

As a result, freeze-dried fruits and vegetables, for example, are now known for their robust nutrient profiles. These foods offer a wide range of vitamins, such as vitamin C and vitamin A, and essential minerals, including potassium and iron. Additionally, they provide antioxidants that are crucial for overall health, such as polyphenols and flavonoids. These advancements ensure that freeze-dried foods remain nutrient-dense, making them valuable components of a balanced diet for weight management.

**2. Flavor and Variety:**

One common misconception about freeze-dried foods is that they may lack flavor or variety. However, the freeze-drying process is continually evolving to enhance the natural taste and texture of foods. Manufacturers are exploring various methods to capture and retain the flavors, colors, and textures that consumers crave.

For instance, freeze-dried fruits can now offer the same burst of sweetness and crunch as their fresh counterparts. The development of new technologies, such as rapid freezing and controlled dehydration, is helping to achieve these improvements. As a result, you can enjoy a wide array of flavors and textures when including freeze-dried foods in your meals and snacks, making them not only nutritious but also appealing and satisfying.

**3. Customized Nutrition:**

The future of freeze-dried foods may involve tailored nutrition to meet individual dietary needs. This advancement aligns with the broader trend of personalized nutrition. With advances in data analysis and artificial intelligence, it's increasingly possible to create customized meal plans that optimize nutrient intake for weight management and overall health.

Imagine a scenario where your dietary preferences, nutritional requirements, and weight management goals are assessed through a smartphone app or a wearable device. This information is then used to generate personalized freeze-dried meal plans. These plans ensure you receive the precise nutrients your body needs while keeping calorie consumption in check. As your goals change, the meal plans can adapt, making it easier to achieve sustainable weight management.

In summary, the advancements in freeze-dried foods are making these options increasingly attractive for weight management and overall well-being. Enhanced nutrition, improved flavor and variety, and the potential for customized nutrition plans are positioning freeze-dried foods as a valuable and convenient resource in the pursuit of a healthy lifestyle. These innovations ensure that freeze-dried foods continue to evolve and meet the diverse needs of individuals seeking effective weight management solutions.

**Section 2: Freeze-Dried Foods and Smart Technology**

The integration of smart technology with freeze-dried foods has the potential to revolutionize the way we approach weight management and healthy living. As technology continues to advance, the combination of freeze-dried foods and smart solutions offers innovative possibilities. In this section, we explore how smart technology can enhance the utilization of freeze-dried foods for weight management:

**1. Personalized Meal Plans:**

Smart technology is poised to analyze your health data, activity levels, and weight management goals to generate personalized freeze-dried meal plans. These plans can be continually adjusted to accommodate your evolving needs. The primary benefits include:

- **Optimal Nutrition:** Smart algorithms can ensure that your meal plans provide the precise nutrients your body requires to meet your weight management and health objectives. This level of customization optimizes your diet for sustainable results.

- **Calorie Control:** By monitoring your calorie intake and expenditure, smart technology can help you maintain your desired calorie balance. Whether your goal is to lose weight, maintain your current weight, or build muscle, personalized meal plans can help you achieve it.

- **Nutritional Diversity:** The algorithms can introduce a wide range of freeze-dried foods into your meal plans, ensuring nutritional diversity. This diversity is essential for receiving a broad spectrum of vitamins, minerals, and antioxidants that support overall well-being.

**2. Nutritional Tracking:**

Mobile apps and wearable devices can incorporate freeze-dried foods into nutritional tracking, simplifying the process of managing your diet. Key advantages of nutritional tracking with freeze-dried foods include:

- **Effortless Monitoring:** By scanning or manually inputting the freeze-dried foods you consume, you can easily track your nutritional intake. These apps can provide real-time feedback on your calorie consumption, macronutrient balance, and the adequacy of your vitamin and mineral intake.

- **Goal Alignment:** Nutritional tracking with smart technology ensures that your dietary choices align with your specific weight management goals. Whether you aim to shed excess weight, maintain your current weight, or build muscle, you can monitor your progress and make informed adjustments.

- **Instant Accountability:** These tools offer immediate accountability, helping you stay on track with your dietary objectives. You can quickly identify areas where you may need to make adjustments and achieve long-term sustainability in your diet.

**3. Smart Kitchen Appliances:**

In the future, kitchen appliances may feature smart technology designed to rehydrate and prepare freeze-dried ingredients with precision. These appliances can transform your home cooking experience by offering the following benefits:

- **Efficiency:** Smart kitchen appliances can make meal preparation more efficient and less labor-intensive. They can precisely control the rehydration process, ensuring that your freeze-dried ingredients are restored to their original textures and flavors.

- **Convenience:** These appliances can simplify the process of incorporating freeze-dried foods into your daily meals. They can automatically select the right rehydration settings, enabling you to prepare delicious, nutritious dishes with ease, even if you have a busy lifestyle.

- **Waste Reduction:** By precisely controlling the rehydration process, smart appliances can minimize waste. You can use only the quantity of freeze-dried ingredients you need, reducing excess and leftover food.

The integration of smart technology with freeze-dried foods offers a future where weight management becomes more precise, convenient, and aligned with your unique needs. Whether it's personalized meal plans, nutritional tracking, or smart kitchen appliances, these technological innovations empower individuals on their weight management journey by simplifying and optimizing their dietary choices.

**Section 3: Sustainability and Environmental Impact**

Sustainability has become a central consideration in our approach to weight management and healthy living. Freeze-dried foods offer several environmental advantages, aligning with the broader goal of creating sustainable and responsible dietary habits. In this section, we explore how the sustainability and environmental impact of freeze-dried foods can influence the future of weight management:

**1. Reduced Food Waste:**

One of the key advantages of freeze-dried foods is their long shelf life, which significantly reduces food waste. Traditional foods often spoil before they can be consumed, resulting in substantial waste at the consumer and supply chain levels. Freeze-dried foods, with their extended shelf life, help mitigate this problem. You can store freeze-dried ingredients for an extended period without worrying about spoilage. This means you're less likely to throw away unused, expired food, which is a common source of waste.

Additionally, freeze-dried foods can help address the issue of excessive food waste in the supply chain. Since freeze-dried ingredients are less perishable, they can be transported and stored more efficiently, reducing waste during the distribution process.

**2. Efficient Resource Use:**

The freeze-drying process is more energy-efficient compared to traditional food preservation methods such as canning or freezing. Traditional methods often involve high temperatures and energy-intensive freezing processes, leading to higher energy consumption and greenhouse gas emissions. In contrast, freeze-drying requires significantly less energy, making it a more eco-friendly preservation method. This efficiency has a positive impact on the environment by reducing energy-related carbon emissions and resource use.

**3. Transportation and Storage:**

Freeze-dried foods are lightweight and compact, which reduces transportation costs and environmental impact. The reduced weight of freeze-dried ingredients means that less fuel is required for shipping, contributing to lower emissions and energy use. Furthermore, their compact size makes them easier to store, which can be particularly valuable in reducing food waste at the consumer level.

Freeze-dried foods are also well-suited for long-term storage. Their resistance to moisture and spoilage ensures that they can be kept for extended periods without the need for refrigeration. This not only saves energy but also reduces the environmental impact associated with the production and operation of refrigeration appliances.

In summary, the sustainability and environmental impact of freeze-dried foods make them an attractive choice for individuals seeking responsible weight management solutions. Their ability to reduce food waste, efficient resource use, and eco-friendly transportation and storage contribute to a healthier planet while supporting your personal weight management and overall wellness goals. As sustainability becomes an increasingly important consideration for individuals and society as a whole, freeze-dried foods offer a practical and responsible approach to weight management.

Chapter 8: Freeze-Dried Foods and the Art of Culinary Innovation

**Section 1: Freeze-Dried Foods in Contemporary Cuisine**

Freeze-dried foods have made a remarkable entry into contemporary cuisine, transforming the way chefs and home cooks approach culinary creation. Their unique attributes, including intense flavors, versatile textures, and vibrant colors, have opened up exciting possibilities for the culinary world. In this section, we explore how freeze-dried foods are influencing and enhancing modern gastronomy:

**1. Flavor Enhancement:**

Freeze-dried foods are prized for their ability to preserve the authentic and concentrated flavors of fresh ingredients. When foods are freeze-dried, they undergo a gentle process that locks in their natural taste. This preservation technique means that the flavors remain vibrant and true to the original, making freeze-dried ingredients a culinary treasure.

Chefs and home cooks alike appreciate the flavor-enhancing qualities of freeze-dried foods. They can incorporate these ingredients to infuse dishes with a burst of flavor, whether it's the sweet intensity of freeze-dried strawberries in a dessert, the savory notes of freeze-dried mushrooms in a risotto, or the zesty kick of freeze-dried herbs in a sauce. Freeze-dried foods serve as natural flavor enhancers, elevating dishes to new levels of deliciousness.

**2. Texture Play:**

The unique textures of freeze-dried ingredients add an element of surprise and excitement to culinary creations. While freeze-drying removes moisture, it preserves the structure of the food, resulting in ingredients that can be either crisp and crunchy or delightfully melt-in-your-mouth.

For instance, freeze-dried fruits like apples and pears provide a satisfying crunch when sprinkled on salads or used as toppings for yogurt or oatmeal. Freeze-dried ice cream retains its characteristic light and airy texture while offering a rich and creamy flavor. The sponge-like quality of freeze-dried sponge cakes can be rehydrated to deliver a unique and indulgent texture. This interplay of textures allows chefs and food enthusiasts to experiment with both taste and mouthfeel, adding a dynamic dimension to their culinary endeavors.

**3. Colorful Creativity:**

The vibrant colors of freeze-dried foods are a visual delight for chefs and those who appreciate beautifully plated dishes. These colors can transform ordinary meals into artistic presentations, adding aesthetic appeal to the culinary experience.

Imagine a bowl of plain oatmeal infused with a burst of crimson freeze-dried strawberries or a salad enlivened by the deep green of freeze-dried spinach. These vibrant hues not only enhance the visual appeal of dishes but also convey a sense of freshness and healthiness. The striking colors of freeze-dried ingredients are instrumental in creating memorable, Instagram-worthy culinary masterpieces.

In contemporary cuisine, freeze-dried foods have emerged as a source of inspiration for chefs and home cooks alike. They have elevated the art of flavor, texture, and presentation, giving rise to a world of culinary creativity that knows no bounds. The intense flavors, versatile textures, and captivating colors of freeze-dried ingredients are essential tools for those seeking to craft extraordinary dining experiences and express their culinary ingenuity.

**Section 2: Fusion of Tradition and Innovation**

Freeze-dried foods represent a fusion of tradition and innovation in the culinary world. They offer a bridge between time-honored cooking techniques and cutting-edge technology, providing chefs and home cooks with a versatile and exciting array of ingredients to work with. In this section, we delve into the ways freeze-dried foods harmoniously blend the best of both culinary worlds:

**1. Enhanced Preservation:**

One of the most significant advantages of freeze-dried foods is their extended shelf life. This preservation technique allows chefs to incorporate seasonal or rare ingredients into their recipes year-round. It's a way to capture the flavors and aromas of peak-season produce or specialty ingredients and extend their presence in the kitchen.

For example, a chef can create a summer-inspired salad in the middle of winter by using freeze-dried strawberries, which maintain the freshness and taste of ripe, sun-ripened berries. This preservation method provides a unique opportunity to bridge the gap between seasonal availability and the desire to create a diverse and dynamic menu throughout the year.

**2. Improved Convenience:**

In a professional kitchen, where time is of the essence, freeze-dried foods provide a level of convenience that is highly valuable. Chefs can access a wide variety of ingredients that might otherwise be challenging to source, prepare, or store. This convenience is particularly useful when working with delicate or perishable ingredients that may be difficult to handle.

Imagine a chef wanting to incorporate fresh herbs into a dish, but they have limited storage space and a tight schedule. Freeze-dried herbs offer a solution. These ingredients are easy to use, require no washing, and eliminate the need to manage perishable herbs. Chefs can access the flavors and aromas of fresh herbs without the added effort or complexity, allowing them to focus on the art of culinary creation.

**3. Unique Applications:**

Freeze-dried foods have sparked unique culinary applications that blend tradition and innovation. Chefs have recognized the potential to manipulate the physical properties of freeze-dried ingredients, which include turning them into powders, infusions, or foams. These innovative uses have opened up new possibilities in culinary artistry.

For instance, freeze-dried fruit powders can be used to intensify the flavor and color of sauces, desserts, or cocktails. They can be incorporated into batters, doughs, and creams to infuse an element of surprise and delight. Additionally, freeze-dried ingredients are used in molecular gastronomy experiments, where their versatile properties come into play in creating captivating culinary experiences.

In the world of gastronomy, the fusion of tradition and innovation is not only encouraged but celebrated. Freeze-dried foods have emerged as a prime example of how culinary traditions can be enhanced with modern techniques. Whether it's the preservation of seasonal flavors, the convenience of accessing unique ingredients, or the exploration of novel culinary applications, freeze-dried foods exemplify the beauty of harmonizing the best of both culinary worlds. This fusion allows chefs to craft extraordinary dishes that respect culinary heritage while embracing the limitless possibilities of the future.

**Section 3: From Home Kitchens to High-End Restaurants**

Freeze-dried foods have transcended the boundaries of professional kitchens and have become equally beloved in the realm of home cooking. At the same time, high-end restaurants are recognizing the versatility and creative potential of freeze-dried ingredients, making them a common feature on both household and fine-dining menus.

**1. Freeze-Dried Foods in Home Kitchens:**

Home cooks are increasingly embracing freeze-dried foods as a valuable addition to their culinary toolkit. There are several reasons for this widespread adoption:

- **Convenience:** Freeze-dried foods offer home cooks a level of convenience that is hard to match. These ingredients are lightweight, easy to store, and have a long shelf life, making them a reliable pantry staple. Home cooks can access a wide range of ingredients, from freeze-dried fruits and vegetables to herbs and spices, allowing them to experiment with flavors and textures without the challenges of sourcing or storing fresh produce.

- **Year-Round Freshness:** Freeze-dried ingredients allow home cooks to enjoy seasonal flavors year-round. Whether it's incorporating freeze-dried strawberries into a winter smoothie or adding freeze-dried herbs to a hearty fall stew, these ingredients offer the opportunity to infuse every season with the tastes of fresh, in-season produce.

- **Exploration and Creativity:** Home cooks are becoming more adventurous in their culinary exploration. Freeze-dried foods provide an avenue for experimentation. The vibrant colors, intense flavors, and unique textures of these ingredients inspire creative dishes and delightful presentations that mirror the artistry found in high-end restaurants.

**2. High-End Restaurants Embracing Freeze-Dried Foods:**

The innovation and versatility of freeze-dried foods have captured the attention of chefs in high-end restaurants. These culinary pioneers are not only incorporating freeze-dried ingredients into their dishes but also pushing the boundaries of what is possible. Here's how high-end restaurants are embracing freeze-dried foods:

- **Creative Expression:** High-end restaurants have long been known for their artistic plating and the use of unusual and rare ingredients. Freeze-dried foods have become a powerful tool for culinary expression, enabling chefs to elevate their creations with intense flavors, vibrant colors, and unique textures.

- **Diverse Menus:** Fine-dining establishments use freeze-dried ingredients to diversify their menus. Chefs can add a touch of novelty and intrigue by introducing seasonal flavors that might otherwise be unavailable, ensuring that diners experience a constantly evolving culinary journey.

- **Molecular Gastronomy:** Freeze-dried ingredients are used in the realm of molecular gastronomy, where chefs deconstruct and reconstruct traditional dishes in imaginative ways. These ingredients can be transformed into foams, powders, and infusions, contributing to the avant-garde nature of high-end cuisine.

In conclusion, freeze-dried foods have permeated both home kitchens and high-end restaurants, reshaping the culinary landscape and offering new horizons for creativity and experimentation. Home cooks are drawn to the convenience and year-round freshness that freeze-dried ingredients provide, while high-end restaurants appreciate the unique attributes of these foods in crafting innovative and visually stunning dishes. The allure of freeze-dried foods is not confined to any one domain, but rather they are celebrated for their capacity to inspire and enrich the art of cooking, regardless of the setting.

Chapter 9: Freeze-Dried Foods and the Future of Nutrition

**Section 1: Addressing Nutritional Gaps**

One of the most pressing challenges in the realm of nutrition is the presence of nutritional gaps in many diets. These gaps often occur due to various factors, including limited access to diverse, fresh foods, dietary restrictions, and lifestyle choices. Freeze-dried foods have emerged as a promising solution to address these nutritional gaps in several ways:

**1. Nutrient-Rich Ingredients:**

Freeze-dried foods, such as fruits, vegetables, and proteins, are inherently nutrient-dense. This means they contain a high concentration of essential vitamins, minerals, and antioxidants that are critical for maintaining health and well-being. These ingredients are not only a convenient addition to meals and snacks but also an effective way to enhance the nutritional content of one's diet.

For instance, freeze-dried fruits like strawberries, blueberries, and mangoes maintain their natural sweetness and a significant portion of their original vitamin C content. Freeze-dried vegetables like spinach, kale, and peas retain their essential vitamins and minerals. Additionally, freeze-dried proteins, such as lean meats or plant-based alternatives, offer high-quality protein without the need for refrigeration. These nutrient-rich ingredients can help individuals bridge the nutritional gaps in their diets, ensuring they receive the essential nutrients they may be missing from other food sources.

**2. Customized Nutrition:**

The future of nutrition is moving towards personalized dietary plans. People are increasingly seeking tailored nutrition solutions that are aligned with their unique health and dietary needs. Freeze-dried foods can play a central role in these personalized plans. The adaptability and versatility of freeze-dried ingredients allow for customized nutrition that caters to individual goals.

Imagine a scenario where a person's dietary preferences, health requirements, and weight management goals are analyzed by a nutrition app. Using this information, the app generates personalized meal plans that incorporate freeze-dried foods to provide the precise nutrients needed. Whether the goal is to lose weight, maintain a balanced diet, or build muscle, these customized plans can help individuals achieve their objectives while ensuring optimal nutrient intake.

As the field of nutritional science continues to advance, the incorporation of freeze-dried foods into personalized nutrition plans can offer a practical and efficient way to meet evolving dietary demands. It not only addresses nutritional gaps but also enhances the overall nutritional quality of one's diet, supporting individuals on their journey toward improved health and well-being.

**Section 2: Sustainable Nutrition**

Sustainability is a growing concern in the field of nutrition and food production. As society becomes more aware of the environmental impact of dietary choices, there is a pressing need for sustainable nutrition solutions. Freeze-dried foods have emerged as a compelling option to promote sustainable dietary practices in the following ways:

**1. Reducing Food Waste:**

Food waste is a significant global issue, contributing to environmental problems and resource depletion. Traditional food preservation methods often fall short in terms of shelf life, leading to the spoilage and disposal of vast quantities of food. Freeze-dried foods, with their extended shelf life, play a crucial role in reducing food waste on multiple fronts:

- **At the Consumer Level:** One of the primary benefits of freeze-dried foods is their ability to remain fresh for an extended period.

Consumers can store these foods without fear of spoilage, which translates to less food waste at home. Freeze-dried ingredients can be used as needed, minimizing the risk of throwing away excess or expired food.

- **In the Supply Chain:** The efficiency of freeze-dried food preservation makes it ideal for reducing food waste in the supply chain. By decreasing spoilage during transportation and storage, freeze-dried ingredients offer a sustainable solution for improving the efficiency of food distribution.

**2. Efficient Resource Use:**

The freeze-drying process is renowned for its efficiency in resource utilization, especially when compared to traditional food preservation techniques like canning or freezing. This efficiency results in several ecological benefits:

- **Energy Consumption:** Freeze-drying requires less energy compared to other methods, as it operates at lower temperatures. This reduction in energy consumption directly translates to a lower environmental impact, particularly in terms of carbon emissions.

- **Resource Conservation:** Traditional food preservation methods can result in high water usage. Freeze-drying, on the other hand, significantly reduces water consumption during food processing. This conservation of resources aligns with sustainability goals, particularly in regions facing water scarcity.

- **Reduction in Waste:** The efficient resource use of freeze-drying extends to the production of freeze-dried ingredients. These ingredients can be prepared in quantities that match demand, minimizing waste associated with excess production and disposal.

Freeze-dried foods are a practical and sustainable solution to address the growing environmental concerns associated with food production and consumption. Their capacity to reduce food waste, minimize energy and resource consumption, and enhance overall efficiency in the food industry contributes to a more sustainable and responsible approach to nutrition, benefiting both individuals and the planet.

**Section 3: Expanding Nutritional Access**

Expanding nutritional access is a pressing global challenge, and freeze-dried foods have the potential to play a significant role in addressing this issue. Whether in disaster relief efforts, humanitarian aid, or futuristic scenarios such as space exploration, freeze-dried foods offer practical solutions to ensure individuals have access to the essential nutrients they need.

**1. Disaster Relief and Humanitarian Aid:**

One of the critical applications of freeze-dried foods is in disaster relief and humanitarian aid efforts. When natural disasters, conflicts, or emergencies strike, access to fresh and nutritious food can become limited. Freeze-dried foods provide an efficient and effective means to meet immediate nutritional needs in crisis situations:

- **Long Shelf Life:** Freeze-dried foods have a long shelf life, ensuring they remain safe and nutritious for extended periods. This feature makes them an ideal choice for stockpiling and distributing food supplies in disaster-prone regions.

- **Lightweight and Compact:** Freeze-dried ingredients are lightweight and compact, making them easy to transport to affected areas. Whether it's sending relief packages by land, air, or sea, the reduced weight and space required by freeze-dried foods enable more efficient delivery.

- **Nutrient-Rich:** These foods are nutrient-dense, which is essential for individuals experiencing the physical and emotional stress of emergencies. They provide a concentrated source of essential vitamins, minerals, and proteins, ensuring that those in need receive adequate nutrition during challenging times.

**2. Space Exploration and Beyond:**

The world of nutrition extends far beyond our planet as humans explore space and consider the possibility of colonizing other celestial bodies. Freeze-dried foods have already found a place in space exploration and hold promise for future extraterrestrial nutrition:

- **Lightweight and Efficient:** Weight and space are precious commodities in space travel, where every ounce of payload makes a difference. Freeze-dried foods are lightweight and compact, making them an efficient choice for space missions. Astronauts can carry a variety of nutrient-rich meals without excessive payload, which is crucial for long-duration missions.

- **Long Shelf Life:** Space missions may span several months or years, and fresh food is not a practical option. Freeze-dried foods provide astronauts with nutritious meals that remain stable and safe for consumption over extended periods. This extended shelf life is crucial for the success and sustainability of space exploration.

- **Sustainability Beyond Earth:** As humanity explores the possibilities of life beyond Earth, freeze-dried foods become a potential source of sustainable nutrition. The efficient preservation and resource use of freeze-drying align with the need for responsible food production and consumption in space environments.

In summary, freeze-dried foods offer innovative solutions for expanding nutritional access in a variety of scenarios. Whether it's in disaster relief, humanitarian aid, or space exploration, these foods provide access to nutrient-rich, lightweight, and long-lasting nutrition. Freeze-dried foods are emblematic of the potential to meet the nutritional needs of diverse populations, even in the most challenging and extraordinary environments.

Chapter 10: Freeze-Dried Foods and the Art of Healthy Living

**Section 1: A Balanced Approach to Healthy Living**

Healthy living is a multi-faceted concept that extends beyond just the absence of illness. It encompasses the physical, mental, emotional, and social aspects of well-being. Nutrition plays a central role in this comprehensive view of health, and freeze-dried foods are positioned as a valuable tool in promoting a balanced approach to healthy living.

**1. Nutrient-Rich Convenience:**

Freeze-dried foods provide a unique combination of nutrient density and convenience. In today's fast-paced world, finding time for meal preparation can be challenging, often leading to dietary choices that prioritize convenience over nutrition. Freeze-dried foods offer a practical solution to this common dilemma:

- **Time Efficiency:** These foods are pre-prepared and lightweight, making them quick and easy to incorporate into meals and snacks. They eliminate the need for extensive washing, chopping, and cooking, saving valuable time.

- **Nutrient Density:** Despite their convenience, freeze-dried foods remain highly nutrient-dense. They retain essential vitamins, minerals, and antioxidants, offering a concentrated source of nourishment. This nutrient density ensures that even quick and simple meals can be rich in vital nutrients, contributing to overall health.

- **Balanced Eating:** Freeze-dried ingredients can be seamlessly integrated into a variety of dietary plans, whether one is following a specific diet, managing weight, or simply seeking to improve nutritional intake. They allow individuals to achieve a balanced diet without the complexity and time investment often associated with healthy eating.

**2. Sustainability as a Lifestyle:**

Sustainability has become a core tenet of a healthy lifestyle. It's about not only personal health but also the health of the planet and future generations. Freeze-dried foods align with the principles of sustainable living, fostering a sustainable lifestyle that incorporates responsible dietary choices:

- **Reducing Food Waste:** One of the primary contributions of freeze-dried foods to sustainability is their ability to reduce food waste. Food waste has significant environmental consequences, from resource depletion to greenhouse gas emissions. By offering long shelf life and minimizing spoilage, freeze-dried ingredients enable individuals to participate in the global effort to reduce food waste.

- **Efficient Resource Use:** The freeze-drying process is inherently resource-efficient. It uses less energy, particularly when compared to traditional preservation methods such as canning or freezing. It also significantly reduces water consumption during food processing. These resource-efficient practices contribute to a more sustainable approach to nutrition.

- **Environmentally Friendly Choices:** By incorporating freeze-dried foods into their diets, individuals are making choices that are kind to the environment. These choices are part of the broader movement toward responsible consumption, promoting the health of the planet alongside personal well-being.

In summary, freeze-dried foods offer a balanced approach to healthy living by combining the convenience required in modern lifestyles with the sustainability principles essential for a holistic view of well-being. These foods empower individuals to make nutritious dietary choices without compromising on time or environmental responsibility. By embracing freeze-dried foods, individuals can cultivate a lifestyle that supports both personal health and the broader goal of a sustainable and thriving planet.

**Section 2: The Power of Food Innovation**

Food innovation plays a pivotal role in reshaping our approach to healthy living, and freeze-dried foods are at the forefront of this transformation. This section explores how the innovative nature of freeze-dried foods contributes to a healthier and more dynamic lifestyle.

**1. Creative Culinary Exploration:**

Healthy living is not merely about consuming the right nutrients; it's also about deriving joy and satisfaction from the foods we eat. Freeze-dried foods have an innate ability to inspire creative culinary exploration and add a sense of adventure to the process of cooking and dining:

- **Exploring Unique Flavors:** Freeze-dried ingredients, with their intense and natural flavors, introduce an exciting dimension to culinary creations. From adding a burst of sweetness to desserts with freeze-dried fruits to enhancing savory dishes with vibrant herbs and spices, these ingredients encourage culinary innovation and experimentation.

- **Texture Play:** The unique texture of freeze-dried foods, which can range from crisp and crunchy to pleasantly melt-in-your-mouth, offers an additional layer of creativity. It allows chefs and home cooks to explore texture contrasts in their dishes, resulting in a more engaging and delightful dining experience.

- **Aesthetic Presentation:** The vibrant colors of freeze-dried foods are visually appealing and add an artistic touch to dishes. The aesthetic appeal of these ingredients is not limited to high-end restaurants; home cooks can also create Instagram-worthy meals, further enhancing the experience of healthy living.

**2. Customized Nutrition:**

The future of healthy living centers around personalized approaches to nutrition. One size does not fit all when it comes to health, and freeze-dried foods play a crucial role in this personalization:

- **Tailored Dietary Plans:** Freeze-dried foods can be seamlessly integrated into personalized dietary plans. Whether someone is following a specific dietary regimen, pursuing weight management, or dealing with specific health requirements, freeze-dried ingredients can be selected to align with these goals.

- **Precise Nutrient Delivery:** Freeze-dried foods offer the advantage of delivering precise nutrients. They enable individuals to meet their unique nutritional needs, whether they require extra protein, specific vitamins, or enhanced mineral intake. This level of precision is fundamental to a customized approach to nutrition.

- **Supporting Healthy Lifestyles:** The adaptability of freeze-dried foods to a variety of dietary preferences, whether plant-based, low-carb, or otherwise, allows individuals to maintain a healthy lifestyle while enjoying the foods they love. It fosters a positive relationship with food and encourages long-term adherence to healthful habits.

In summary, freeze-dried foods exemplify the power of food innovation in promoting a healthier and more dynamic lifestyle. They inspire creative culinary exploration, encourage a personalized approach to nutrition, and add vibrancy and excitement to healthy living. By embracing the innovation inherent in freeze-dried ingredients, individuals can enhance their well-being while savoring the pleasures of culinary creativity and customized nutrition.

**Section 3: Promoting Wellness Beyond the Plate**

Healthy living encompasses not only the nutritional aspects of well-being but also the broader implications of our dietary choices on personal resilience, environmental stewardship, and the quality of life. Freeze-dried foods have the power to impact wellness beyond the plate in several meaningful ways.

**1. Preparedness and Resilience:**

Healthy living extends to preparedness for unexpected challenges and the ability to respond with resilience. In this context, freeze-dried foods offer important advantages:

- **Food Security:** In a world where natural disasters, emergencies, and unexpected crises can disrupt food supply chains, having a stock of freeze-dried foods provides a level of food security. Individuals and communities are better prepared to face unforeseen challenges by having access to reliable and long-lasting nutrition.

- **Long Shelf Life:** The extended shelf life of freeze-dried foods ensures that they remain safe and nutritious for extended periods. This feature is vital for maintaining food supplies in emergency scenarios, ensuring that individuals and families have access to sustenance during difficult times.

- **Adaptation and Resilience:** The ability to adapt to unforeseen challenges and rebound from adversity is a fundamental aspect of healthy living. Freeze-dried foods enable individuals and communities to adapt and build resilience in the face of unexpected disruptions to the food supply, which ultimately contributes to a healthier and more secure way of life.

**2. Environmental Stewardship:**

A healthy lifestyle is closely linked to environmental stewardship, as the health of the planet is intricately connected to personal well-being. Freeze-dried foods encourage eco-friendly choices and responsible consumption:

- **Reducing Food Waste:** One of the most significant environmental contributions of freeze-dried foods is their capacity to reduce food waste. Food waste has far-reaching consequences, from resource depletion to environmental degradation. By offering long shelf life and minimizing spoilage, freeze-dried ingredients enable individuals to play a role in reducing food waste, thereby supporting a more sustainable planet.

- **Efficient Resource Use:** The freeze-drying process is inherently resource-efficient. It uses less energy and water compared to other preservation methods, which reduces its environmental impact. The choice to incorporate freeze-dried foods into one's diet aligns with the global movement toward resource-efficient and eco-friendly practices.

- **Promoting Sustainable Living:** Freeze-dried foods empower individuals to make sustainable choices in their daily lives. These choices include not only nutrition but also the responsible use of resources and the reduction of their ecological footprint. By making environmentally conscious dietary choices, individuals contribute to a healthier world and set an example for future generations.

**3. Exploration and Imagination:**

Wellness is not only about physical health but also about nurturing the mind and spirit. Freeze-dried foods encourage a sense of exploration and imagination:

- **Culinary Exploration:** The unique properties of freeze-dried ingredients inspire creative culinary exploration. The act of creating new dishes, exploring unique flavors and textures, and presenting visually stunning meals enhances the overall enjoyment of food and fosters a deeper connection to the culinary arts.

- **Lifestyle Creativity:** Beyond the culinary realm, freeze-dried foods encourage creative thinking and lifestyle experimentation. Whether it's creating meal plans, designing sustainable living strategies, or finding innovative solutions for unexpected challenges, freeze-dried foods provide a platform for a more imaginative and fulfilling way of life.

In conclusion, freeze-dried foods offer transformative potential by promoting wellness beyond the plate. They support preparedness and resilience in the face of adversity, align with principles of environmental stewardship, and inspire exploration and imagination. By embracing freeze-dried foods, individuals can experience a holistic approach to healthy living that extends to personal resilience, environmental responsibility, and the joyful exploration of life's possibilities.

Chapter 11: Staying Committed and Motivated

**Section 1: Strategies to Maintain Long-Term Weight Loss**

While losing weight is a significant achievement, the ultimate goal is to maintain that weight loss over the long term. This section delves into effective strategies to help you sustain your weight loss, ensuring that your hard-earned progress becomes a permanent part of your healthier lifestyle.

**1. Consistent Eating Habits:**

Consistency in your eating habits is crucial to maintaining weight loss. This means adopting a stable and balanced diet that you can sustain over time. Here are key points to consider:

- **Balanced Nutrition:** Continue to prioritize a well-balanced diet rich in essential nutrients. Include a variety of fruits, vegetables, lean proteins, whole grains, and healthy fats in your daily meals. A balanced diet provides the necessary nutrients for overall health and helps you avoid nutrient deficiencies.

- **Mindful Eating:** Stay mindful of portion sizes and eating behaviors. Avoid overindulging or consuming large portions, which can lead to weight regain. Mindful eating involves paying attention to hunger and fullness cues, savoring each bite, and avoiding emotional eating.

- **Avoiding Trigger Foods:** Identify trigger foods that may lead to overeating and consider limiting or avoiding them. This could include highly processed, calorie-dense, or sugar-laden items that have previously contributed to weight gain.

- **Meal Planning:** Planning your meals and snacks in advance can help you make healthier choices. Having a plan reduces the likelihood of impulsive, less nutritious food choices. Consider preparing your meals at home, as this gives you more control over ingredients and portion sizes.

**2. Regular Physical Activity:**

Physical activity is not only essential for weight loss but also for maintaining your weight. Here's how to incorporate regular physical activity into your routine:

- **Set Realistic Exercise Goals:** Establish realistic and achievable exercise goals. This might involve aiming for a certain number of weekly workouts, increasing the duration or intensity of your exercise over time, or trying new physical activities that you enjoy.

- **Diverse Workouts:** Incorporate a variety of exercises to prevent monotony and avoid plateaus. Combining cardiovascular exercises, strength training, and flexibility routines can help you stay engaged and maintain your fitness levels.

- **Consistency is Key:** Commit to a regular exercise routine that you can realistically maintain. Consistency is more important than intensity. Even if your workouts are not extremely vigorous, the cumulative effect of regular activity is what matters most.

- **Adaptive Exercise:** Be prepared to adapt your exercise routine to your evolving needs and circumstances. Life can be unpredictable, but adjusting your workouts to fit your schedule, health status, and changing goals ensures you continue to prioritize physical activity.

**3. Monitor Your Progress:**

Ongoing monitoring of your progress is critical to prevent weight regain and stay on track:

- **Regular Weigh-Ins:** Periodic weigh-ins can help you detect any signs of weight regain early. If you notice a slight increase in your weight, you can take action to address it before it becomes a significant issue.

- **Food Diary and Mobile Apps:** Keeping a food diary or using mobile apps that track your meals and nutritional intake can be an effective way to stay accountable. These tools also offer insight into your dietary patterns and habits.

- **Consultation with Professionals:** Consider periodic consultations with healthcare professionals or nutritionists. They can provide valuable guidance and support, review your progress, and offer tailored advice to help you maintain your weight loss.

- **Mental and Emotional Well-Being:** Don't overlook the mental and emotional aspects of your weight maintenance journey. Stay attuned to your emotional relationship with food and seek counseling or support groups if needed.

By applying these strategies, you can work towards the long-term maintenance of your weight loss. Remember that this is a journey, and setbacks may occur. The key is to approach them with resilience and the knowledge that you have the tools and strategies to continue progressing toward your health and wellness goals.

**Section 2: Setting Realistic Goals and Tracking Progress**

Maintaining your weight loss over the long term requires not only commitment and motivation but also setting achievable goals and tracking your progress effectively. This section delves into the importance of goal-setting and monitoring to ensure that your weight loss remains sustainable.

**1. S.M.A.R.T. Goals:**

Setting S.M.A.R.T. (Specific, Measurable, Achievable, Relevant, Time-bound) goals is a fundamental aspect of maintaining your weight loss:

- **Specific:** Clearly define your goals. Instead of a vague goal like "I want to maintain my weight loss," specify what you want to achieve. For example, "I aim to maintain my current weight within a range of plus or minus three pounds."

- **Measurable:** Goals should be quantifiable so you can track your progress. You need to know when you've achieved them. For instance, you could measure success by keeping your weight within a certain range or by exercising a set number of days per week.

- **Achievable:** Your goals should be attainable. Ensure they are realistic for your lifestyle, health, and time constraints. Unrealistic goals can lead to frustration and reduced motivation.

- **Relevant:** Your goals should be relevant to your long-term health and wellness. They should align with your personal values and reflect what is most meaningful to you in your weight maintenance journey.

- **Time-bound:** Set a timeframe for achieving your goals. This provides a sense of urgency and helps you stay focused. For example, "I want to maintain my weight within a range of plus or minus three pounds for the next six months."

**2. Keep a Journal:**

Maintaining a journal can be a powerful tool in tracking your progress. Consider these aspects of journaling:

- **Food Diary:** Recording what you eat and drink daily helps you become more aware of your dietary choices. This practice also allows you to identify patterns or triggers that may lead to overeating or unhealthy choices.

- **Exercise Log:** Keep track of your physical activity, including the type, duration, and intensity of workouts. An exercise log helps you monitor your commitment to regular physical activity and assess your progress.

- **Emotional Record:** Keeping a record of your emotions and feelings in your journal can help you understand your relationship with food. Emotional eating can undermine weight maintenance, and identifying emotional triggers is the first step in addressing this issue.

**3. Celebrate Milestones:**

Acknowledging your achievements and celebrating milestones is crucial for maintaining motivation and a sense of accomplishment:

- **Non-Scale Victories:** Not all victories are measured by the scale. Non-scale victories might include fitting into an old pair of jeans, receiving compliments on your appearance, or having more energy and stamina.

- **Small Wins:** Celebrate small victories along the way. Achieving these short-term goals can boost your confidence and motivation. Reward yourself for reaching milestones such as consistently meeting your exercise goals, preparing a week's worth of balanced meals, or reducing your waist size.

**4. Visualize Success:**

The power of visualization should not be underestimated. Imagining your success can provide motivation and help you stay committed:

- **Mental Imagery:** Take time to visualize yourself achieving your goals. Picture how it will feel to maintain your weight loss and the benefits that come with it. This mental imagery can boost your motivation and resilience when faced with challenges.

By setting realistic goals, keeping a detailed journal, celebrating your achievements, and using visualization techniques, you can effectively track your progress and maintain your weight loss. These practices help keep you accountable, focused, and motivated throughout your long-term weight maintenance journey.

**Section 3: Finding Motivation and Support in Your Journey**

Staying motivated and finding support is crucial in the journey of maintaining long-term weight loss. This section explores various strategies and resources to help you stay committed and inspired as you continue your path towards a healthier lifestyle.

**1. Identify Personal Motivators:**

Understanding your personal motivations is fundamental to maintaining weight loss. These motivations provide the fuel to keep you committed and focused on your goals:

- **Health and Well-Being:** Many people are motivated by the desire to improve their overall health and well-being. This includes reducing the risk of chronic diseases, improving cardiovascular health, and enhancing overall vitality.

- **Increased Energy:** Weight loss often results in increased energy levels. This newfound vitality can be a powerful motivator for staying committed, as it allows you to engage more fully in your daily life and activities.

- **Enhanced Confidence:** Achieving weight loss goals can boost self-confidence. The realization that you can set and achieve significant goals in your life can serve as a powerful motivator to continue leading a healthier lifestyle.

- **Participation in Activities:** Some individuals are motivated by their desire to participate in activities they may not have been able to before their weight loss. Whether it's hiking, running, or playing sports, having new opportunities for physical activities can be a strong driving force.

- **Improved Quality of Life:** Ultimately, maintaining weight loss contributes to an improved quality of life. This can encompass many aspects, from better sleep and improved relationships to increased job opportunities and the ability to engage in new hobbies.

**2. Seek Social Support:**

Engaging with a supportive network of friends, family, or like-minded individuals can be a powerful tool for motivation. Here's how to find and leverage social support:

- **Support Groups:** Consider joining weight loss support groups or forums, either in-person or online. These communities offer a space for sharing experiences, advice, and encouragement with others who are on similar journeys.

- **Friend and Family Involvement:** Involve your friends and family in your journey. Share your goals, challenges, and successes with them. Having a supportive network can provide you with motivation and accountability.

- **Accountability Partners:** Partner with a friend or family member to act as an accountability partner. You can set goals together, exercise together, and check in with each other regularly. This mutual support can keep you both motivated.

**3. Visualize Success:**

Mental imagery can serve as a powerful motivator:

- **Visualize Your Future:** Take time to visualize your future self as someone who has successfully maintained their weight loss. Picture yourself living a vibrant and healthy life, enjoying your favorite activities, and feeling confident in your appearance.

- **Create a Vision Board:** Some people find creating a vision board with images, quotes, and reminders of their goals and motivations to be a helpful tool for staying inspired and focused.

- **Review Your Progress:** Regularly review your progress and remind yourself of how far you've come. This reflection can provide motivation and encouragement to continue your journey.

**4. Stay Informed:**

Staying informed about health and wellness topics can renew your commitment to a healthy lifestyle:

- **Read and Learn:** Continue to educate yourself about nutrition, fitness, and well-being. Knowledge is a powerful motivator and can inspire you to make informed and health-conscious choices.

- **Stay Updated:** Keep abreast of the latest research and developments in health and wellness. Being aware of new findings and trends can guide your decision-making.

By identifying your personal motivators, seeking social support, visualizing your success, and staying informed, you can bolster your commitment to maintaining long-term weight loss. Remember that motivation can ebb and flow, but these strategies offer a well-rounded approach to help you stay on track and continue to lead a healthy and fulfilling life.

Chapter 12: Beyond Weight Loss – Maintain a Healthy Lifestyle

**Section 1: Transitioning from Weight Loss to Weight Maintenance**

The transition from a phase of active weight loss to one of weight maintenance is a pivotal moment in your journey toward a healthier lifestyle. During this phase, your focus shifts from creating a caloric deficit to sustainably balancing your energy intake and expenditure. This section provides guidance on making this transition effectively.

**1. Gradual Adjustments:**

As you reach your weight loss goal, it's important to make gradual adjustments to your eating and exercise habits. The abrupt cessation of a strict diet can lead to weight regain. Instead, ease into a maintenance phase:

- **Caloric Adjustments:** Gradually increase your caloric intake to meet your maintenance needs. This prevents your body from perceiving sudden energy deficits, which could trigger hunger and cravings. Start by adding a small number of calories each week until you reach your maintenance level.

- **Physical Activity:** Maintain your regular exercise routine but consider shifting the focus from primarily calorie burning to overall fitness and well-being. This might involve incorporating strength training, flexibility exercises, or other fitness goals.

- **Mindful Eating:** Continue to practice mindful eating. Mindfulness helps you stay in tune with your body's hunger and fullness cues, preventing overeating. Eating mindfully can also help you savor your meals and make healthier food choices.

**2. Monitor and Adapt:**

Consistent monitoring and adaptation are key during the transition phase:

- **Regular Check-Ins:** Continue to monitor your weight regularly. It's essential to notice any significant fluctuations early to address them effectively. If you notice weight gain or loss outside your target range, take action promptly.

- **Food Diary:** Maintain a food diary, even if you're no longer actively dieting. This practice helps you remain aware of your dietary choices and identify any patterns that could lead to weight regain.

- **Emotional Eating Awareness:** Stay vigilant about emotional eating patterns. Stress, emotional triggers, or changes in your daily routine can influence your relationship with food. Identifying these patterns enables you to address them and make healthier choices.

- **Adaptation:** Be prepared to adapt your habits as necessary. Life is dynamic, and what works for you one month may need to be adjusted the next. When you encounter changes in your schedule, stress levels, or other factors, be flexible in your approach to maintain your weight.

**3. Sustainable Habits:**

The habits that led to your successful weight loss should not be abandoned once you've reached your goal. They form the foundation for sustainable weight maintenance:

- **Balanced Diet:** Continue to prioritize a balanced diet that includes a variety of fruits, vegetables, lean proteins, whole grains, and healthy fats. This dietary approach is not only for weight loss but also for long-term well-being.

- **Regular Physical Activity:** Physical activity should remain a part of your daily life. Exercise is essential for maintaining not only your weight but also your overall health, fitness, and vitality.

- **Positive Mindset:** Cultivate a positive mindset. Your attitude toward your lifestyle change is crucial. Focus on the benefits you've gained from your weight loss journey, such as improved health, increased energy, and a sense of accomplishment.

In summary, the transition from weight loss to weight maintenance is a critical phase in your journey toward lifelong health. Making gradual adjustments, monitoring your progress, and adapting to changes in your life are essential steps. Maintaining sustainable habits, including a balanced diet, regular exercise, and a positive mindset, is key to ensuring your long-term success in maintaining a healthy lifestyle.

**Section 2: Incorporating Freeze-Dried Foods into a Sustainable, Healthy Eating Plan**

Freeze-dried foods are a valuable resource in the journey to maintaining a healthy lifestyle. They offer convenience, nutrition, and versatility, making them an excellent addition to your long-term eating plan. This section explores how to incorporate freeze-dried foods into your diet for sustained well-being.

**1. Nutrient-Packed Convenience:**

Freeze-dried foods are nutrient-dense and convenient. Here's how to make the most of these benefits:

- **Balanced Meals:** Incorporate freeze-dried fruits, vegetables, and proteins into your daily meals. These ingredients add essential vitamins, minerals, and protein without compromising on nutrition. For instance, adding freeze-dried berries to your breakfast cereal or freeze-dried peas to your salads ensures you get a variety of nutrients.

- **Healthy Snacking:** Freeze-dried snacks, such as fruits and vegetables, are a smart choice for between-meal cravings. They're easy to pack, require no refrigeration, and provide a satisfying crunch while offering a nutrient boost.

- **Emergency Preparedness:** Keep a stock of freeze-dried foods for emergencies or unexpected situations. They have a long shelf life and can serve as a reliable source of nutrition during times when fresh foods may not be available.

**2. Minimizing Food Waste:**

Minimizing food waste is an important aspect of a sustainable eating plan. Freeze-dried foods contribute to this goal:

- **Extended Shelf Life:** One of the standout features of freeze-dried foods is their extended shelf life. Unlike fresh produce that can spoil quickly, freeze-dried ingredients remain safe and nutritious for extended periods. This attribute minimizes food waste in your kitchen.

- **Portion Control:** Freeze-dried foods often come in portion-controlled packaging, which reduces overconsumption. This can be especially helpful for weight maintenance by helping you avoid overeating.

- **Zero Food Spoilage:** Freeze-dried foods don't spoil, which means you won't have to throw away rotten or expired items. This minimizes the environmental impact of food waste.

**3. Culinary Exploration:**

Experimenting with freeze-dried foods can add variety and excitement to your meals:

- **Texture and Flavor:** Freeze-dried ingredients offer unique textures and intense flavors. For example, adding freeze-dried pineapple to a stir-fry or freeze-dried corn to soups can elevate your dishes, making healthy eating more enjoyable.

- **Creative Recipes:** Explore creative recipes that feature freeze-dried ingredients. This can involve making homemade granola bars with freeze-dried fruits or crafting colorful smoothie bowls with freeze-dried berry toppings. These inventive meals make healthy eating fun.

- **Visual Appeal:** The vibrant colors of freeze-dried fruits and vegetables can enhance the visual appeal of your dishes. Aesthetically pleasing meals are more likely to be enjoyed, making it easier to adhere to a healthy eating plan.

By incorporating freeze-dried foods into your long-term eating plan, you not only enhance the convenience of your diet but also minimize food waste and add creativity and variety to your meals. Freeze-dried ingredients are versatile, nutritious, and offer culinary exploration, making them a valuable addition to your ongoing journey toward a healthier lifestyle.

**Section 3: Strategies for Lifelong Wellness**

Achieving and maintaining a healthy lifestyle is a long-term commitment that goes beyond weight loss and dietary choices. This section delves into the strategies necessary for lifelong wellness, encompassing physical, emotional, and mental well-being.

**1. Goal Setting:**

Setting and regularly reassessing your health and wellness goals is essential for staying motivated and maintaining your well-being over the long term:

- **Clear Objectives:** Your goals should be clear and specific. These goals can range from physical achievements like running a marathon, to emotional objectives such as reducing stress or improving self-confidence.

- **Adaptation:** Life is dynamic, and so are your goals. As your circumstances and priorities change, be willing to adapt your goals to align with your evolving desires and needs.

- **Short and Long-Term:** Consider both short-term and long-term goals. Short-term goals can offer quick victories, while long-term goals provide a sense of purpose and direction.

**2. Self-Care:**

Prioritizing self-care is essential for lifelong wellness. Self-care encompasses practices that nurture your mental, emotional, and physical health:

- **Stress Management:** Implement effective stress management techniques, whether it's through mindfulness, meditation, yoga, or other relaxation practices. Reducing stress is crucial for overall well-being.

- **Adequate Sleep:** Ensure you get enough quality sleep. A well-rested body and mind are better equipped to handle daily challenges and maintain good health.

- **Emotional Health:** Focus on your emotional health. This includes recognizing your emotions, seeking support or counseling when needed, and cultivating emotional resilience.

**3. Regular Check-Ins:**

Regular check-ins with healthcare professionals, nutritionists, and personal trainers are valuable for maintaining lifelong wellness:

- **Health Screenings:** Schedule regular health check-ups, screenings, and tests to detect any potential issues early. Prevention and early intervention are key to long-term well-being.

- **Nutritional Guidance:** Continue to seek nutritional guidance and advice from professionals to ensure you're making informed choices about your diet and maintaining balanced nutrition.

- **Physical Activity Support:** Consult with personal trainers or fitness experts for exercise plans and guidance. They can help you adapt your workout routines to your evolving fitness goals and needs.

**4. Variety in Activities:**

Variety in physical activities is essential for keeping your fitness routine exciting and sustainable:

- **Try New Activities:** Experiment with different forms of exercise and physical activities. Exploring new sports, classes, or recreational activities can keep your routine fresh and enjoyable.

- **Cross-Training:** Incorporate cross-training to balance your fitness regimen. It can help prevent overuse injuries, promote overall fitness, and keep you engaged in your workouts.

**5. Emotional Health:**

Pay attention to your emotional well-being, as it plays a vital role in lifelong wellness:

- **Mindfulness and Meditation:** Engage in mindfulness practices and meditation to foster emotional awareness and well-being. These practices can help you manage stress, reduce anxiety, and improve emotional resilience.

- **Emotional Support:** Don't hesitate to seek emotional support when needed. Talking to a therapist, counselor, or support group can provide valuable guidance and coping strategies.

**6. Mindful Eating:**

Continue to practice mindful eating, as it forms a healthy relationship with food:

- **Portion Control:** Maintain control over your portion sizes and avoid overeating. Mindful eating techniques help you savor your meals and reduce the likelihood of mindless consumption.

- **Meal Planning:** Continue to plan your meals ahead of time. Meal planning ensures you make balanced, healthful choices and reduces the temptation to eat unhealthy options.

**7. Community Engagement:**

Engaging with your community or social networks contributes to a sense of belonging and support:

- **Share Your Journey:** Share your wellness journey with friends, family, or your community. This can foster a sense of connection, inspire others, and hold you accountable.

- **Group Activities:** Participate in group activities, fitness classes, or community events. Engaging in social activities adds enjoyment to your wellness routine and strengthens your social bonds.

In conclusion, maintaining lifelong wellness involves a holistic approach to physical, emotional, and mental health. Setting clear goals, prioritizing self-care, seeking professional guidance, and practicing mindfulness are all essential aspects of your wellness journey. By integrating these strategies into your daily life, you can ensure that you not only achieve your wellness goals but maintain a state of well-being and vitality for the long term.

Chapter 13: Conclusion - Your Lifelong Journey to Health

The concluding chapter of your journey to a healthier lifestyle reflects on your achievements and reinforces the principles and insights you've gained throughout this book. It encapsulates the idea that the pursuit of well-being is a lifelong journey, rather than a finite destination.

**1. Celebrating Success:**

Begin by celebrating your achievements. Whether you've shed excess pounds, improved your fitness, or enhanced your overall well-being, these milestones are worth acknowledging. Take pride in your accomplishments and use them as motivation to continue striving for a healthier life.

**2. Acknowledging Challenges:**

Recognize that your journey was not without its share of challenges. There were likely moments of doubt, hurdles to overcome, and the occasional setback. These challenges are a natural part of the process, and acknowledging them as learning opportunities will fortify your resilience.

**3. Embracing Lifelong Learning:**

View your journey as an ongoing process of self-improvement. The pursuit of health is not a destination but a journey marked by continuous learning. Stay curious and open to new information, emerging trends, and evolving best practices in the fields of nutrition, fitness, and overall wellness.

**4. Staying Motivated:**

Maintaining motivation is key to sustaining your healthy lifestyle. You'll find that motivation may ebb and flow over time. During periods of lower motivation, revisit your reasons for embarking on this journey. Remember the benefits you've experienced, such as improved energy, self-confidence, and well-being.

**5. Setting New Goals:**

As you move forward, continue to set new goals. These can encompass various aspects of your health, including physical fitness, emotional well-being, and personal growth. Setting and achieving new objectives keeps your journey fresh and exciting.

**6. Finding Balance:**

In your pursuit of well-being, strive to find balance in all areas of your life. This balance includes managing your time, maintaining a sense of equilibrium between work and personal life, and creating space for relaxation and self-care.

**7. Building a Support Network:**

Your support network is an invaluable asset. Maintain your connections with friends, family, and communities that encourage and inspire you in your journey. Whether in person or through virtual support groups, these connections provide the motivation and accountability you need.

**8. Nurturing Emotional Health:**

Recognize the profound connection between emotional and physical well-being. Emotional health is a cornerstone of your overall health. Practice stress management, emotional awareness, and self-compassion as you navigate the challenges of daily life.

**9. Staying Mindful:**

Continue to practice mindful eating and mindful living. Being present in the moment helps you make healthier choices and fosters a deeper appreciation for the simple pleasures in life.

**10. Reflecting on Freeze-Dried Foods:**

As you conclude your journey, consider how freeze-dried foods have become a reliable and healthful component of your diet. Whether in the form of nutrient-dense snacks, ingredients for balanced meals, or emergency provisions, these foods have added a layer of convenience and sustainability to your lifestyle.

**11. Paying It Forward:**

Share your experiences and knowledge with others. You have valuable insights and practical strategies to offer those who may be at the beginning of their own wellness journeys. Act as a source of inspiration and guidance for your friends, family, and community.

**12. Embracing the Journey:**

Remember that your pursuit of well-being is not a destination but a lifelong journey. Embrace each day as an opportunity to make choices that enhance your physical and emotional health. By focusing on the process rather than the outcome, you'll find lasting fulfillment and sustained well-being.

In conclusion, your journey to health is a continuous process marked by growth, adaptation, and transformation. The principles you've embraced – from balanced nutrition and regular exercise to emotional wellness and a sense of community – will serve as your guiding compass. Keep moving forward, stay curious, and embrace the lifelong adventure that is your pursuit of health and well-being.

Additional Resources

This chapter provides you with a wealth of additional resources to enhance your journey toward a healthier lifestyle, with a particular focus on freeze-dried foods, support, and tools for weight loss and nutrition tracking.

**1. Freeze-Dried Food Brands and Suppliers:**

- **Thrive Life:** Thrive Life offers a wide variety of freeze-dried foods, including fruits, vegetables, meats, and dairy products. Their products are designed for long-term storage and everyday use.

- **My Patriot Supply:** This supplier specializes in emergency preparedness foods, offering freeze-dried fruits, vegetables, and complete meals with a focus on sustainability and shelf life.

- **Augason Farms:** Augason Farms is known for its long-term food storage options, including freeze-dried foods. They provide a range of products suitable for everyday consumption.

- **Valley Food Storage:** This supplier offers freeze-dried meals, fruits, and vegetables, with an emphasis on providing nutritious and flavorful options for long-term storage or daily use.

**2. Additional Reading, Websites, and Communities:**

- **Dietary Guidelines for Americans:** The official government resource provides comprehensive guidance on nutrition, diet, and health.

- **American Heart Association:** Their website offers valuable resources on heart-healthy eating and lifestyle choices.

- **Eat Right:** This website is run by the Academy of Nutrition and Dietetics, offering credible information on nutrition and healthy eating.

- **SparkPeople:** An online community that provides support, recipes, and fitness resources for individuals on their health journey.

- **Reddit Weight Loss Communities:** Subreddits like r/loseit and r/1200isplenty offer supportive communities where you can share experiences, get advice, and find motivation.

**3. Tools and Apps for Weight Loss and Nutrition Tracking:**

- **MyFitnessPal:** A popular app for tracking calories, exercise, and nutrition. It offers a vast database of foods and user-friendly features.

- **Lose It!:** This app helps you set weight loss goals, track your food intake, and monitor your progress. It also includes a barcode scanner for convenience.

- **Cronometer:** A comprehensive nutrition tracking app that provides detailed information on your micronutrient intake.

- **Fitbit:** Not only is it a wearable for tracking activity and sleep, but the Fitbit app also allows you to log your food and water intake, set goals, and monitor your weight.

- **MyPlate by Livestrong:** An app that provides calorie and nutrition tracking, recipes, and fitness tips.

- **Nutrition Facts:** An app that lets you scan barcodes to get detailed nutrition information about packaged foods.

- **Happy Scale:** This app focuses on weight tracking and smoothing out weight fluctuations to provide a more accurate view of your progress.

- **Yazio:** A user-friendly app for tracking calories, macros, and exercise. It also offers personalized meal plans and recipes.

These additional resources are valuable tools to support your ongoing journey to a healthier lifestyle. From finding reputable freeze-dried food suppliers to accessing reliable information, support communities, and apps for weight loss and nutrition tracking, these resources will help you stay on the path to improved health and well-being.

Chapter 14: Conclusion

In this concluding chapter, we'll recap the numerous advantages of freeze-dried foods for weight loss and offer some final words of encouragement and advice for a healthier, happier you.

**1. Summing up the Benefits of Freeze-Dried Foods for Weight Loss:**

Throughout this book, you've learned about the remarkable benefits of freeze-dried foods in your journey to weight loss:

- **Nutrient Retention:** Freeze-drying preserves the essential nutrients in foods, ensuring you get maximum nutrition without added calories.

- **Long Shelf Life:** Freeze-dried foods have an extended shelf life, making them a sustainable option that minimizes food waste.

- **Convenience:** These foods are lightweight, easy to store, and require no refrigeration, making them perfect for on-the-go, busy schedules, or emergency preparedness.

- **Portion Control:** Many freeze-dried foods come in portion-controlled packaging, helping you maintain portion control, a crucial aspect of weight management.

- **Variety and Versatility:** Freeze-dried fruits, vegetables, and proteins add variety and flavor to your diet, making healthy eating more enjoyable and sustainable.

- **Reduced Food Cravings:** The concentrated flavors and textures of freeze-dried foods can help satisfy cravings without overindulgence.

**2. Encouragement and Final Words of Advice for a Healthier, Happier You:**

As you continue on your journey to a healthier, happier you, remember these key pieces of advice:

- **Celebrate Your Achievements:** Celebrate the milestones you've reached. Recognize the hard work and dedication you've put into your health and well-being.

- **Acknowledge Challenges:** Acknowledge that challenges and setbacks are part of the process. They're opportunities for growth and learning.

- **Keep Learning:** Wellness is an ongoing journey, not a destination. Continue to seek knowledge and stay open to new information and practices.

- **Stay Motivated:** Maintaining motivation is key to lasting success. Revisit your reasons for embarking on this journey, and consider setting new goals to keep your motivation high.

- **Set New Goals:** Keep setting new objectives in different aspects of your life. These goals will keep you engaged and excited about your journey.

- **Find Balance:** Strive to find balance in all areas of your life, from work to personal time. Prioritize relaxation and self-care.

- **Build a Support Network:** Your support network is a vital asset. Lean on friends, family, and communities that offer encouragement and motivation.

- **Nurture Emotional Health:** Emotional well-being is intertwined with physical health. Practice stress management, emotional awareness, and self-compassion.

- **Stay Mindful:** Continue practicing mindful eating and living. Being present in the moment can lead to healthier choices and greater appreciation for life's simple pleasures.

- **Embrace the Journey:** Remember that the pursuit of well-being is an ongoing journey, not a finite destination. Embrace each day as an opportunity to make choices that enhance your physical and emotional health.

In conclusion, freeze-dried foods have proven to be an invaluable resource on your path to weight loss and a healthier lifestyle. Their benefits, including nutrient retention, convenience, and long shelf life, have added a layer of sustainability and nutrition to your journey. As you move forward, continue to embrace the journey toward a healthier, happier you, celebrating your achievements, acknowledging your challenges, and setting new goals. By staying motivated and maintaining a supportive network, nurturing emotional health, and practicing mindfulness, you'll find lasting fulfillment and well-being on your lifelong journey to health.

**Index**

**A**

- **Achievements (Chapter 14):**

    - Celebrating, [14.1]
- **Additional Resources (Chapter 13):**
    - Apps for weight loss and nutrition tracking, [13.3]
    - Conclusion (Chapter 14), [14]
    - Emotional wellness and stress management, [13.2]
    - Freeze-dried food brands and suppliers, [13.1]
    - Nutrition tracking and weight loss, [13.3]
    - Recommendations, [13.1]
- **Adaptation (Chapter 12):**
    - Gradual adjustments, [12.1]
    - Strategies for lifelong wellness, [12.3]
- **Balance (Chapter 12):**
    - Finding, [12.6]
- **Benefits (Chapter 14):**
    - Freeze-dried foods for weight loss, [14.1]
    - Summing up, [14.1]
- **Building a Support Network (Chapter 12):**
    - Engaging with communities, [12.7]
- **C**

- **Celebrating Achievements (Chapter 14):**
    - [14.1]
- **Conclusion (Chapter 14):**
    - [14]
    - Benefits of freeze-dried foods for weight loss, [14.1]
    - Encouragement and final words of advice, [14.2]
- **Culinary Exploration (Chapter 12):**
    - Creative recipes, [12.3]
- **D**

- **Diet in Weight Management (Chapter 1):**
    - Role of diet, [1.2]
- **E**

- **Emotional Health (Chapter 12):**
    - Emotional support, [12.5]

  - Mindfulness and meditation, [12.5]
- **Encouragement (Chapter 14):**
  - Final words of advice, [14.2]
- **F**

- **Finding Balance (Chapter 12):**
  - [12.6]
- **Freeze-Dried Foods (Chapter 2):**
  - Common misconceptions, [2.3]
  - How freeze-drying works, [2.1]
- **G**

- **Goal Setting (Chapter 12):**
  - Short and long-term goals, [12.1]
- **Gradual Adjustments (Chapter 12):**
  - [12.1]
- **H**

- **Healthy Lifestyle (Chapter 13):**
  - Strategies for lifelong wellness, [13.3]
- **I**

- **Index, [Index]**
- **Introducing Freeze-Dried Foods (Chapter 1):**
  - [1.3]
- **L**

- **Learning (Chapter 14):**
  - Keep learning, [14.3]
- **Maintaining Motivation (Chapter 12):**
  - [12.4]
- **Mindful Eating (Chapter 12):**
  - [12.6]
- **Mindset (Chapter 12):**
  - Positive mindset, [12.3]
- **Motivated (Chapter 11):**

- Staying motivated, [11.1]
- **N**

- **Nutrient-Packed Convenience (Chapter 12):**
  - [12.2]
- **Nutritional Value (Chapter 3):**
  - Comparing the nutritional content, [3.1]
  - Freeze-drying preserves essential nutrients, [3.2]
  - Role of freeze-dried fruits, vegetables, and proteins, [3.3]
- **P**

- **Portion Control (Chapter 14):**
  - [14.1]
- **Practical Strategies (Chapter 12):**
  - [12.2]
- **Preparation (Chapter 2):**
  - How freeze-drying works, [2.1]
- **R**

- **Reflection (Chapter 12):**
  - [12.7]
- **Resources (Chapter 13):**
  - Additional reading, websites, and communities, [13.2]
  - Freeze-dried food brands and suppliers, [13.1]
  - Index, [Index]
  - Tools and apps for weight loss and nutrition tracking, [13.3]
- **Role of Diet in Weight Management (Chapter 1):**
  - [1.2]
- **S**

- **Self-Care (Chapter 12):**
  - [12.2]
- **Setting New Goals (Chapter 14):**
  - [14.2]
- **Stress Management (Chapter 12):**
  - [12.4]

- **Support Network (Chapter 12):**
  - [12.7]
- **Sustainable Habits (Chapter 12):**
  - [12.4]
- **T**

- **Tracking Progress (Chapter 11):**
  - [11.2]

**References**

- **Campbell, T. Colin. (2005). The China Study. BenBella Books.**

- **Brown, Brené. (2012). Daring Greatly. Penguin.**

- **Pollan, Michael. (2006). The Omnivore's Dilemma. Penguin.**

- **Pollan, Michael. (2008). In Defense of Food. Penguin.**

- **[Official Dietary Guidelines for Americans. (2020). U.S. Department of Health and Human Services.](https://www.dietaryguidelines.gov/)**

- **[American Heart Association. (n.d.).](https://www.heart.org/en)**

- **[Eat Right (Academy of Nutrition and Dietetics). (n.d.).](https://www.eatright.org/)**

- **[SparkPeople. (n.d.).](https://www.sparkpeople.com/)**

- **[Reddit Weight Loss Communities. (n.d.).](https://www.reddit.com/r/loseit/)**

- **[Fitbit. (n.d.).](https://www.fitbit.com/global/us/home

RECIPES

Certainly! Here are ten delicious freeze-dried food recipes that are easy to prepare and perfect for various occasions:

**1. Freeze-Dried Fruit Parfait:**

- 1 cup of freeze-dried mixed berries
- 1 cup of vanilla Greek yogurt
- 1/4 cup of granola
- Honey (optional)

  Directions: In a bowl, layer the freeze-dried fruits, yogurt, and granola. Drizzle with honey if desired. Enjoy a nutritious and quick parfait.

**2. Freeze-Dried Veggie Stir-Fry:**

- 1 cup of freeze-dried mixed vegetables (rehydrated)
- 1 cup of cooked rice
- 2 tablespoons of stir-fry sauce
- 1 tablespoon of vegetable oil

  Directions: Heat the oil in a pan, add the rehydrated vegetables and stir-fry for a few minutes. Add the cooked rice and stir-fry sauce. Cook until heated through and serve.

**3. Creamy Tomato Soup:**

- 1 cup of freeze-dried tomato chunks
- 2 cups of hot water
- 1/2 cup of heavy cream
- Salt and pepper to taste

  Directions: Combine the tomato chunks and hot water in a pot. Let it sit for a few minutes until rehydrated. Blend the mixture until smooth, add heavy cream, and season with salt and pepper. Heat before serving.

**4. Southwest Black Bean Salad:**

- 1 cup of freeze-dried black beans (rehydrated)
- 1 cup of corn kernels
- 1/2 cup of freeze-dried bell peppers (rehydrated)
- 1/4 cup of diced red onion
- 2 tablespoons of lime juice
- 1 tablespoon of olive oil
- 1 teaspoon of chili powder
- Salt and pepper to taste

Directions: In a large bowl, combine rehydrated black beans, corn, bell peppers, and red onion. In a separate bowl, whisk together lime juice, olive oil, chili powder, salt, and pepper. Drizzle the dressing over the salad and toss gently.

**5. Backpacker's Omelette:**

- 1/2 cup of freeze-dried scrambled eggs (rehydrated)
- 1/4 cup of freeze-dried spinach (rehydrated)
- 2 tablespoons of freeze-dried mushrooms (rehydrated)
- 1 tablespoon of grated cheese (optional)
- Salt and pepper to taste

Directions: Heat a non-stick pan and add the rehydrated eggs, spinach, and mushrooms. Cook until the omelette sets, sprinkle with cheese if desired, fold in half, and serve.

**6. Mediterranean Pasta Salad:**

- 1 cup of freeze-dried penne pasta (rehydrated)
- 1/2 cup of freeze-dried cherry tomatoes (rehydrated)
- 1/4 cup of freeze-dried cucumber (rehydrated)

- 1/4 cup of sliced olives
- 2 tablespoons of olive oil
- 1 tablespoon of balsamic vinegar
- 1/2 teaspoon of dried oregano
- Salt and pepper to taste

Directions: In a large bowl, combine rehydrated pasta, cherry tomatoes, cucumber, and olives. In a separate bowl, whisk together olive oil, balsamic vinegar, oregano, salt, and pepper. Drizzle the dressing over the pasta salad and toss gently.

**7. Sweet and Spicy Beef Jerky:**

- 1 cup of freeze-dried beef strips (rehydrated)
- 1/4 cup of soy sauce
- 2 tablespoons of honey
- 1/2 teaspoon of chili flakes
- 1/2 teaspoon of garlic powder
- 1/2 teaspoon of ginger powder

Directions: In a bowl, combine the soy sauce, honey, chili flakes, garlic powder, and ginger powder. Add the rehydrated beef strips and marinate for at least 30 minutes. Lay the beef strips on a baking sheet and bake at a low temperature (170°F or 75°C) until dried, approximately 3-4 hours.

**8. Cheesy Broccoli Rice:**

- 1 cup of freeze-dried broccoli (rehydrated)
- 1 cup of cooked rice
- 1/2 cup of shredded cheddar cheese
- 2 tablespoons of butter
- Salt and pepper to taste

Directions: In a pan, melt the butter and add the rehydrated broccoli. Cook for a few minutes, then stir in the cooked rice and shredded cheddar cheese. Cook until the cheese melts and season with salt and pepper.

**9. Chia Seed Pudding:**

- 2 tablespoons of chia seeds
- 1 cup of freeze-dried mixed berries (rehydrated)
- 1 cup of almond milk (or your choice of milk)
- 1 tablespoon of honey (optional)

Directions: Mix chia seeds and almond milk in a jar or bowl. Stir well, cover, and refrigerate overnight. In the morning, layer the chia pudding with rehydrated mixed berries and drizzle with honey if desired.

**10. Crunchy Granola Bars:**

- 1 cup of freeze-dried mixed nuts (rehydrated)
- 1 cup of freeze-dried mixed fruits (rehydrated)
- 2 cups of rolled oats
- 1/2 cup of honey
- 1/4 cup of peanut butter
- 1/4 cup of chocolate chips (optional)

Directions: In a large bowl, mix rehydrated nuts, rehydrated fruits, rolled oats, honey, and peanut butter. Stir in chocolate chips if desired. Press the mixture into a baking dish and refrigerate until firm. Cut into bars and enjoy.

**11. Creamy Chicken and Vegetable Pasta:**

- 1 cup of freeze-dried chicken (rehydrated)
- 1 cup of freeze-dried mixed vegetables (rehydrated)
- 1 cup of pasta
- 1/2 cup of heavy cream

- 1/4 cup of grated Parmesan cheese
- 2 tablespoons of butter
- Salt and pepper to taste

1. Cook the pasta according to the package instructions and set aside.
2. In a large pan, melt the butter over medium heat.
3. Add the rehydrated chicken and cook until browned.
4. Add the rehydrated mixed vegetables and sauté for a few minutes.
5. Stir in the heavy cream and grated Parmesan cheese. Cook until the sauce thickens.
6. Season with salt and pepper.
7. Toss the cooked pasta in the creamy sauce and serve hot.


**12. Freeze-Dried Apple Cinnamon Oatmeal:**

- 1 cup of freeze-dried apple slices (rehydrated)
- 1/2 cup of rolled oats
- 1 cup of water
- 1/4 cup of milk (or a milk substitute)
- 1 teaspoon of cinnamon
- 1 tablespoon of honey
- Chopped nuts (optional)

1. In a bowl, combine rehydrated apple slices, rolled oats, and water.
2. Microwave for 2-3 minutes, stirring occasionally until the oats are cooked and the mixture thickens.
3. Stir in milk, cinnamon, and honey.
4. Top with chopped nuts if desired and enjoy.


**13. Thai Peanut Noodles:**

- 1 cup of freeze-dried tofu (rehydrated)
- 1 cup of freeze-dried bell peppers (rehydrated)
- 1 cup of rice noodles
- 1/4 cup of peanut sauce
- Chopped peanuts for garnish
- Fresh cilantro leaves for garnish
- Lime wedges for serving

1. Cook the rice noodles according to the package instructions and set aside.
2. In a large pan, combine rehydrated tofu and bell peppers.
3. Add the peanut sauce and heat until everything is well coated.
4. Serve the peanut tofu mixture over the cooked rice noodles.
5. Garnish with chopped peanuts, fresh cilantro, and lime wedges.


**14. Freeze-Dried Pineapple Chicken Skewers:**

- 1 cup of freeze-dried chicken (rehydrated)
- 1 cup of freeze-dried pineapple chunks (rehydrated)
- 2 tablespoons of soy sauce
- 1 tablespoon of honey
- 1/2 teaspoon of ginger powder
- Skewers for grilling

1. In a bowl, mix the rehydrated chicken, rehydrated pineapple chunks, soy sauce, honey, and ginger powder.
2. Thread the chicken and pineapple onto skewers.
3. Grill the skewers until the chicken is cooked and slightly charred.
4. Serve hot.


**15. Lemon Zest Freeze-Dried Shrimp:**

- 1 cup of freeze-dried shrimp (rehydrated)
- Zest of one lemon

- 2 tablespoons of olive oil
- 2 cloves of garlic, minced
- 1/4 teaspoon of red pepper flakes (optional)
- Fresh parsley for garnish

1. In a pan, heat olive oil over medium-high heat.
2. Add the rehydrated shrimp and cook for a few minutes until heated through.
3. Stir in lemon zest, minced garlic, and red pepper flakes.
4. Cook for an additional minute.
5. Garnish with fresh parsley and serve.


**16. Mediterranean Quinoa Salad:**

- 1 cup of freeze-dried quinoa (rehydrated)
- 1/2 cup of freeze-dried cherry tomatoes (rehydrated)
- 1/4 cup of freeze-dried cucumber (rehydrated)
- 1/4 cup of Kalamata olives
- 2 tablespoons of feta cheese
- 2 tablespoons of olive oil
- 1 tablespoon of red wine vinegar
- Fresh basil leaves for garnish

1. In a large bowl, combine rehydrated quinoa, cherry tomatoes, cucumber, olives, and feta cheese.
2. In a small bowl, whisk together olive oil and red wine vinegar. Drizzle over the salad.
3. Toss to combine and garnish with fresh basil leaves.


**17. Berry Bliss Smoothie:**

- 1 cup of freeze-dried mixed berries (rehydrated)
- 1 cup of yogurt (or a yogurt substitute)
- 1/2 cup of milk (or a milk substitute)

- 1 banana
- 1 tablespoon of honey
- Chia seeds (optional)

1. In a blender, combine rehydrated mixed berries, yogurt, milk, banana, and honey.
2. Blend until smooth.
3. Pour into a glass, garnish with chia seeds if desired, and enjoy.


**18. Italian Caprese Salad:**

- 1 cup of freeze-dried mozzarella cheese (rehydrated)
- 1 cup of freeze-dried cherry tomatoes (rehydrated)
- 1/4 cup of freeze-dried basil leaves (rehydrated)
- 2 tablespoons of balsamic vinegar
- 2 tablespoons of olive oil
- Salt and pepper to taste

1. In a bowl, combine rehydrated mozzarella cheese, cherry tomatoes, and basil leaves.
2. Drizzle with balsamic vinegar and olive oil.
3. Season with salt and pepper.
4. Toss to combine and serve.


**19. Vegetarian Minestrone Soup:**

- 1 cup of freeze-dried mixed vegetables (rehydrated)
- 1/2 cup of freeze-dried pasta
- 1/4 cup of freeze-dried kidney beans (rehydrated)
- 1/4 cup of freeze-dried green beans (rehydrated)
- 1/4 cup of freeze-dried zucchini (rehydrated)
- 2 cups of vegetable broth
- 1 teaspoon of Italian seasoning
- Grated Parmesan cheese for garnish

1. In a pot, combine rehydrated mixed vegetables, pasta, kidney beans, green beans, zucchini, vegetable broth, and Italian seasoning.
2. Bring to a boil, then reduce the heat and simmer until the pasta and vegetables are tender.
3. Season with salt and pepper.
4. Serve hot with grated Parmesan cheese on top.


**20. Lemon Blueberry Muffins:**

- 1 cup of freeze-dried blueberries (rehydrated)
- 2 cups of all-purpose flour
- 1/2 cup of sugar
- 2 teaspoons of baking powder
- 1/2 teaspoon of salt
- 1/2 cup of milk
- 1/4 cup of melted butter
- Zest of one lemon
- 2 eggs

1. Preheat the oven to 375°F (190°C) and line a muffin tin with paper liners.
2. In a bowl, combine rehydrated blueberries, flour, sugar, baking powder, and salt.
3. In another bowl, mix milk, melted butter, lemon zest, and eggs.
4. Combine the wet and dry ingredients, stirring until just combined.
5. Spoon the batter into the muffin cups.
6. Bake for 20-25 minutes, or until a toothpick comes out clean.
7. Allow the muffins to cool before serving.


These freeze-dried food recipes offer a range of flavors and dishes, from savory pasta to sweet muffins. Enjoy exploring these culinary options and making the most of the convenience and nutrition that freeze-dried ingredients provide.

Enjoy these delicious and convenient freeze-dried food recipes!